THE AGING SPINE

THE AGING SPINE

Water Exercise & Treatment Principles

By Martha White

Foreword by John West, P.T.
and Chapter by
Howard Cotler, M.D.

iUniverse, Inc.
New York Lincoln Shanghai

THE AGING SPINE
Water Exercise & Treatment Principles

iUniverse, Inc.

For information address:
iUniverse, Inc.
2021 Pine Lake Road, Suite 100
Lincoln, NE 68512
www.iuniverse.com

THIS BOOK IS NOT A SUBSTITUTION FOR MEDICAL ADVICE. PLEASE CONSULT YOUR DOCTOR BEFORE BEGINNING AN EXERCISE PROGRAM.

ISBN: 0-595-32887-3

Printed in the United States of America

"Although the disc has historically played a major role as a mediator of low back pain, nearly every other structure in the low back has also been shown to be a potential source of pain."

—Porterfield and DeRosa 1991, 11

Contents

ACKNOWLEDGEMENTS

I have had tremendous support from my co-workers and patients the past two years as this book has come together. I must acknowledge some tremendous mentors I have worked with over the years: Martin Blacker, M.D., a brilliant physician and pioneer in pain management programming in Houston; the late Roy Don Wilson, A.T.C., an extremely talented leader and dynamic athletic trainer; John West, P.T., a legend in the Houston physical therapy scene, a brilliant businessman and compassionate therapist; and Dr. Howard Cotler, an excellent spine surgeon and dedicated physician. I owe most of my thanks however to Mark Brandt, who helped me organize my book and my thoughts. Truly, this book could not have come to pass without him.

This book is dedicated to my family: Jordan, Katie, and Lisa.

PREFACE

There is a tremendous amount of information on back pain that is released annually for the general public, the health professional and physician, and researchers. With each surge of information, new techniques in the care and management of back pain emerge and the means of intervention improve.

In most cases, there is not a definitive cause of back pain; many times there may be a combination of problems that are causing the pain and disability. It is frustrating for the patient, the doctor and adjunct health care personnel as everyone searches for effective intervention. The focus of the book is on common degenerative processes of the spine. Granted, this is a small piece in the large scope of back pain but it focuses on the most common types of back problems. The intent of the book is to give an overview of the pertinent anatomy as it relates to the degenerative process. The overview is targeted primarily for the lay public and is therefore general, with the intent to introduce material but not overwhelm the reader. Thanks to the internet, more in depth information is available for those seeking it.

It is my hope that the reader will learn something that will help him better understand his back pain, and learn techniques that will assist in more effective pain management. It's about learning to live more harmoniously with back pain. When you better understand what you're dealing with, it is possible, but it is a learned process.

FOREWORD

Martha White has done it again. She has given us another book that is easy to understand and identifies in a factual and non-biased form why most of us have back pain and what to do for it.

This book confirms all my beliefs regarding care of the spine. Estimates are that 70% of adults suffer from back pain at some time in their lives and that over $26 billion is spent each year on back pain with most of this going to a small percent who never get better. It is no wonder that payers are up in arms at who to pay and what to pay.

The focus of Martha's book solves this problem by telling you what to do for yourself. Her book confirms my belief that your back is only as good as your last workout. There is no saving account there. You have to do the work and you must be consistent.

Her 20 years of providing care to such patients has given her a plethora of experience on how to provide proper programs for individual problems. Her explanations are cogent and understandable. This book is a must read for those of us who have experienced back pain and for those of us who want to prevent it.

John D. West, P.T.

Houston, Texas

INTRODUCTION

Miserable. Burning. Dull. Aching. Unrelenting. Sharp. Numb. I can't live this way. Just shoot me! I have heard all of these comments over the years when I've asked someone to describe their low back pain. Welcome to the club of BACK PAIN; everyone is a reluctant member.

Eight out of 10 individuals will suffer from low back pain in their lifetime. Many may suffer an isolated episode of back pain after "overdoing it" or having a little fender bender. Most of us, however, fall into another category. Chronic back pain is defined as back pain lasting longer than five months. This book touches on both categories of back pain, but specifically addresses chronic back pain.

For years, the standard treatment of back pain was moist heat, ultrasound, massage and Williams Flexion exercises (knee(s)-to-chest), along with pain medication. This regime would go on indefinitely. "Indefinitely" here means there was not the Big Brother scrutiny of insurance companies and HMOs that now exists. "Indefinitely" was also the norm because research had not yet proven how ineffective passive physical therapy treatments of heat, ultrasound, massage were on a **long term** basis in the treatment of low back pain, and how much more effective specific exercises were as a means of intervention. "Cure me today" is what every back patient thinks when he walks into his doctor's or therapist's office for the first time. "If I can just get rid of this pain, I can get back to my life." Everyone is looking for some kind of magic. Much more is required of patients today in the successful management of back pain. "It is thought if the pain is taken away, function automatically returns. In most cases, these approaches are temporary solutions, at best, because the patient is not taught how to manage his own problem." (Porterfield and DeRosa 1991, 2)

If you fall into the category of chronic low back pain (greater than five months), you are going to have to learn techniques and lifestyle modification to live a functional life. "Functional" means an uninterrupted life—maybe not pain-free, but a life that is (1) not keeping you out of or off work, (2) isolated from friends and family, (3) prescription drug dependent. Basically, you are not functional if you are unable to do simple things like cooking, grocery shopping, sitting through meetings, or attending your child's ballgame or concert. I know you; you walk through my door everyday.

There are effective treatment approaches out there, but they require the active participation of the patient. Showing up at the clinic or doctor's office to have something "done to you" has proven itself ineffective for any type of long-term intervention with back pain. Within the guidelines of safety and comfort, appropriate exercise is the answer and a major part of the overall equation. Whether this exercise is to prevent surgery or as a means of recovery after surgery, it is integral.

The onset of back pain doesn't just suddenly occur, with the exception of isolated trauma like a fall or car accident. In most cases, it has been an insidious, ongoing process of wear and tear over a period of time. It may be job related, postural or structural (degenerative bony changes), but it finally manifests in some fashion as low back pain. Perhaps it is degenerative disc disease, spinal stenosis or osteoarthritis. This ongoing erosive process may also result in a bulging or herniated disc. The manifestation of back pain may be predominantly one type of degenerative category, or a combination of degenerative problems. More often it is a combination of degenerative processes that result in low back pain and disability. Rarely is low back pain black and white, but instead, many shades of gray.

Degenerative Changes of the Spine

ANATOMY

"Joints function to move; muscles contract and generate tension; ligaments restrain."

—(DeFranca 1996, 135)

The body is a work of art in its design and operation. There are many checks and balances built into the system to keep it running as smoothly as possible, for as long as possible. The physiological checks and balances are numerous and beyond the scope of this book.

To understand your type of back pain, you first need to understand what is going on with the spine and the anatomical structures involved. Let's review the basic structures of the spine and their functions before going into the specific degenerative processes that occur with the spine. As we get more specific, we will include research from spinal specialists, but first things first.

The Spinal Column

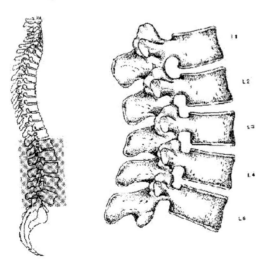

Reprinted from *Clinical Anatomy of the Lumbar Spine and Sacrum*, 3rd Edition, Nikolai Bogduk, 2, Copyright (1997), with permission from Elsevier.

The spinal column is divided into three sections. The uppermost portion is the cervical spine, the middle portion is comprised of the thoracic spine that is attached to the rib cage, and the lumbar spine which rests upon the fused, wedge-shaped bone called the sacrum. The sacrum sits at an approximate angle of 45 degrees. This angle slightly increases with standing and even more so in the wearing of high heels, which tilts the pelvis slightly forward. This explains why a day or evening in high heels could result in a flare-up of back pain.

The spinal column consists of three curves, one curve slightly forward in the cervical spine, and one lower curve in the thoracic spine, which is more posterior. The lowest curve is located in the lumbar spine and curves forward. The "S" shaped design of the spine helps it better function and load like a spring or coil.

"There is a mechanical basis for these normal anatomic curves; they give the spinal column increased flexibility and augmented, shock-absorbing capacity, while at the same time maintaining adequate stiffness and stability at each inter-vertebral joint level." (White and Panjabi 1978, 2) Joints located in between each individual vertebra are called facet joints. These joints "provide a bony interlock-ing mechanism that resists forward displacement." (Bogduk 1997, 57) There is also extensive ligamentous attachments throughout the spine, but more so between the lumbar spine and pelvis. This ligamentous support provides a great deal of stability and safeguards the spinal cord from injury. They can also con-tribute to some of the degenerative changes the spine undergoes that ultimately alter the mechanics and efficiency of spinal mobility and function, as you will later see. Muscles also provide tremendous checks and balances to the spine.

"The spine with its ligaments intact but devoid of muscles is an extremely unstable structure." (White and Panjabi 1978, 47) All of these structures are inte-gral to the checks and balances of the spine. We have seen how the loose "S" design of the spine balances the body from the head to toes. This design also allows for the spine to take on additional pressures and equally distribute them throughout the spine, protecting it from injury. The spinal cord is enclosed in the bony canal of the spinal column, and adequately encapsulated from injury, with the exception of tremendous external trauma, for example, diving accidents or car accidents. These traumas are of high velocity, sudden impact; in these incidences the capacity of bone, ligament and muscle is overwhelmed and unable to accom-modate the forces thrust upon it.

I don't want to bog down too much in the anatomy; we are more interested in how all of these systems work together. Once the actual functional relationships are disrupted, the degenerative process begins. Let's look at those relationships more closely. "Abnormalities of function occur first and lead later on to structural abnormalities." (Kirkaldy-Willis 1983, 23)

The spine consists of thirty-three individual vertebrae. The cervical spine (neck) consists of 7 vertebrae; the thoracic spine consists of 12 vertebrae that are attached to the rib cage, and the lumbar spine has 5 vertebrae that sit on top of a wedge-shaped fused bone called the sacrum. The sacrum has 5 fused bones and the coccyx (or "tail bone") has 4 small mobile segments. The sacrum fits down in between the 2 ilium, which make up the pelvis. The three principle functions of the vertebrae are: 1) protect the spinal cord, 2) provide rigidity, and 3) allow mobility. (Grelsamer and Loebl 1997, 171)

The cervical vertebrae support the head and allow for bending, rotating, flexing and extending. The thoracic vertebrae are attached to a rib on either side and this design lends itself to more rigidity. There is limited motion in flexion (bending) and rotation. The rib cage increases the stability of the thoracic portion of the spine by limiting motion. "This is why it exhibits fewer osteoarthritic changes and fewer disc problems." (Grelsamer and Loebl 1997, 175)

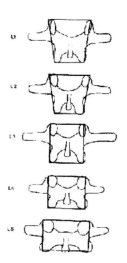

The design of the lumbar spine is related to its function. These vertebrae are larger than the cervical and thoracic vertebrae due to the heavier loads they must bear. Each lumbar vertebrae progressively bears more weight than the vertebrae above it. The fifth lumbar vertebra bears the greatest load and the rectangular design provides a wider base to support this. The fourth and fifth lumbar vertebrae bear greater loads and allow for more motion than the other lumbar vertebrae. The fourth and fifth lumbar vertebrae account for the highest degree of degeneration, about 90%. Surgery is most common at these two levels of the lumbar spine. Reprinted from *Clinical Anatomy of the Lumbar Spine and Sacrum*, 3rd Edition, Nikolai Bogduk, 229, Copyright (1997), with permission from Elsevier.

"The size and mass of the vertebrae increases from the first cervical to the last (lumbar) vertebrae. This is a mechanical adaptation to the progressively increasing loads."

—(White and Panjabi 1978, 23)

Discs

Discs are located in between each spinal vertebra and provide the shock absorption of the spine. This function accommodates added loads or pressures to the spine. These additional pressures may come from external loads, such as carrying a box, child or pet, or from sustained postures.

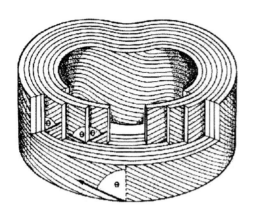

The outer part of the disc is made up of densely woven rings that are fiberous in nature; these are called annulus fibrosus. The rings are angled in design and alternate in direction every other ring. The annular rings are 60% to 70% water and are densely packed with collagen to make it a turgid, relatively stiff body. "In all movements, the annulus fibrosus acts like a ligament to restrain movements and stabilize the (vertebral) joint to some degree. All fibers resist distraction and all are involved in weight-bearing." (Bogduk 1997, 30) Reprinted from *Clinical Anatomy of the Lumbar Spine and Sacrum*, 3rd Edition, Nikolai Bogduk, 15, Copyright (1997), with permission from Elsevier.

Later we will look at the degenerative process of the disc and see how it sometimes starts from the innermost portion and works its way outward. If you look at the illustration, you see how the fibers of one annular ring run in one direction, while the next ring has fibers that run in the opposite direction. This design helps the stability of the disc and spine as it accommodates loads over the duration of a lifetime. This design also guards the integrity of the disc against strong rotational pressures that may come from work related tasks, sports or activities of daily living, to a lesser degree.

The center of the disc is called the nucleus pulposus; an oval shaped gelatinous base. The water content of the nucleus ranges from 70% to 90%. "The nucleus pulposus allows for binding large amounts of water. The water content increases the resilience of the entire disc. The elastic intervertebral discs ease the loads that weigh on the spine and distribute them in a manner that the pressure exerted on any one portion of the vertebrae is minimized." (Grelsamer and Loebl 1997, 172) As we age, the water content of the disc decreases along with the shock absorption capacity of the spine. Just like a car with worn shocks, we take bumps a lot harder and recover slower as we get older. The primary purpose of the water-based nucleus is the displacement of additional pressures through the disc and spinal column, regardless of the source. This function of the disc protects us from sudden, unexpected loads, like a fall or car accident. If injury does occur, the force simply was greater than the tissue's capacity to protect.

Facet Joints

The facet joints of the spine, also known as the zygapophysial joints, are the bony articular joints between each vertebra. These are responsible for the smooth translation of movement throughout the spinal column. "The facets, vertebral bodies and the discs work together as a functional unit that allows for forces to be transferred through the (lumbar) spine." (Porterfield and DeRosa 1991, 84)

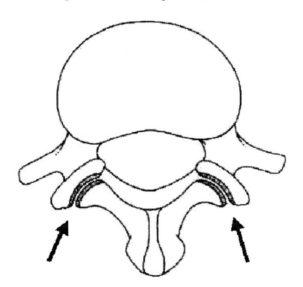

The facet joints enable the vertebra to move upon one another and protect each individual vertebrae from forward and rotational displacement. These interlocking joints are covered by a cartilaginous sheet that allows the bony surfaces to move smoothly. Sometimes the cartilaginous surfaces lock up as one goes from a flexed posture to upright, like rising from a seated position. These joints and the cartilaginous surfaces erode from trauma and aging. The capsule surface can thicken through ingrowth, impairing the joint mechanics. Bony spurring can develop around these joints as well. The facet joints are located on each side of the individual vertebrae throughout the entire spine. There are twice as many facet joints versus vertebrae in the spinal column. Reprinted from *Clinical Anatomy of the Lumbar Spine and Sacrum*, 3rd Edition, Nikolai Bogduk, 34, Copyright (1997), with permission from Elsevier.

"Where bones articulate with each other, there is a smooth cartilage lining that secretes lubricating fluid. The function of the facet joint is to guide and limit the motion of the vertebrae." (Goldstein 1995, 134) We have looked broadly at the spine and the way it functions. The vertebrae are a weight bearing body. The disc, which is composed of annular rings and a pulposus center, is responsible for the equal distribution and displacement of any additional pressures to the spine.

These extra loads may come from a change in posture (sitting or climbing stairs), or from external loads like carrying a child, a box, a suitcase or bag.

DEGENERATIVE PROCESSES OF THE SPINE

With some exceptions, the back works well and we feel invincible until that first episode of back pain hits and we know its something more than muscle strain. This time the injury may linger for days or longer. The injury doesn't have to be dramatic, like moving a large piece of furniture by yourself.

> When my first big episode of back pain hit, I was in great shape and jogging daily. That morning, I simply turned and leaned over to my right and felt immediate pain; I couldn't straighten up. I did all I could do—I lay in bed all weekend. Getting off my feet allowed that inflamed joint or disc to recover, and I returned to work Monday. I also resumed jogging, writing off the incident as isolated. I soon forgot all about it, but the damage was done. I was 27 years old at the time.

The degenerative process typically manifests between the mid-twenties to the late-forties. I said "manifests;" remember, the degenerative process has already started and it's now beginning to express itself. Let's now look closer at specific degenerative processes of the spine. Remember back pain is not black and white, but shades of gray.

Degenerative Spinal Processes

> *"The intervertebral disc, between the ages of 30 and 50 years, is changing from one of a rather healthy, resilient, high water content to a relatively dry, scarred disc characteristic of individuals over 50."*
>
> —(White and Panjabi 1978, 281)

"My spine is degenerating," said my patient, an attractive forty-five year old mother. She was answering another of my aquatic patients, a newcomer who was making small talk. "Oh, my goodness," said my older patient, making a face as she turned away. I turned away too, slightly shaking my head. It's not as catastrophic as it sounds. Everyone's spine is degenerating! It's not a disease, but an aging process. "If only people knew these things about their backs," I thought, then the term "degenerative disc disease" wouldn't be so unnerving.

Degenerative Disc Disease

"Degenerative spine" is not an exclusive club; in fact, everyone is eventually a member. Degenerative changes, whether in the disc itself or the facets, the articulating joints of the spine, will eventually appear and demand attention. Let's look at what is actually happening with the disc once it lets its presence be known.

"Cracks and cavities may develop which enlarge to become clefts and overt fissures." (Bogduk 1997, 173) When I was taking a course on a particular technique in back care called the McKenzie Method, I had a great teacher that broke this process down quite eloquently. The instructor, Shelia McBride, PT, put it this way. Think of the nucleus (center) of the disc as a body of water, say a river. With aging, traumatic injuries, whatever the source, the annular rings around the disc begin to break down. Think of this as little tributaries developing off of that large contained body of water. It gets harder and harder to maintain the integrity of the nucleus and surrounding annular rings. As this happens, the nucleus (central body of water) becomes less organized and begins to dry out.

"Less able to attract water, these discs take longer to resume their original configuration and structure after deformation." (Bogduk 1997, 175) With significant traumas from falls, accidents, sports or work related tasks, your discs sustain physical breakdown of tissue, which heal and then lay down scar tissue. The scar tissue is not as elastic, so with the next bout of work-related tasks or exercise, micro-trauma may again appear, and it will appear at the point of least resistance, which will probably be the site of scar tissue. When you push your back too hard, as evidenced by a lingering backache, you are sustaining micro-trauma to the discs, facet joints and other components of the spinal segment.

> I kept trying to jog after injuring my back. I could complete the 3 to 4 mile jog, but the quality was lacking. Then that dull backache and stiffness would set in within the next 4 hours. I kept trying this over and over, until finally I realized it wasn't worth it. Not only was my back not getting any better, it was gradually getting worse.

Is it wrong to "test the waters" every so often and see where you are with your back? Not necessarily and you'll do it anyway. But, if your response to the test is a lingering backache for the next several days, as mine was, I'd say the task is too much for your low back. The discs, facets and all components of the spinal unit cannot meet the physical demands required of that task. At this point, you don't have the capacity, tissue and joint-wise, to perform that task (or sport) consistently without sustaining some degree of micro-trauma along the way.

"Internal disc disruption is a condition in which the internal architecture of the disc is disrupted but its external surface remains the same. The probability of the disc becoming painful therefore increases the further the fissure extends into the annulus." (Bogduk 1997, 207) English translation. What this fine researcher, Nikolai Bogduk, is saying is that as the nucleus, the center of the disc, begins to break down, you develop tears and fissures in the fibrous rings surrounding the nucleus. These tears and fissures come from aging and micro-traumas over the years. This process takes place over a period of years and may also be job related. There is a gradual migration of material from the inner nucleus of the disc to the outer annular rings. Remember the angular crisscross design of the annular rings? The design itself helps retard the overall degenerative process.

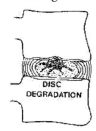

DISC DEGRADATION

Reprinted from *Clinical Anatomy of the Lumbar Spine and Sacrum,* 3rd Edition, Nikolai Bogduk, 211, Copyright (1997), with permission from Elsevier. "If two-thirds of the annulus were disrupted by a fissure, the intact fibers in the remaining one-third would be exposed to three times their accustomed stress." (Bogduk 1997, 207) This scenario can lead to isolated episodes of back pain that become more cyclic in nature. In some instances however, further stresses may lead to herniation, where the nucleus pulposus finally breaks through the outermost annular rings. Disc herniation is known as herniated nucleus pulposus (HNP).

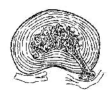

"Less able to bind water, the nucleus is less able to sustain pressures. In time, the annulus buckles under this load and the disc loses height, which compromises the functions of all joints in this affected vertebral segment." (Bogduk 1997, 211) This doesn't mean you are going to end up with a herniated disc. It does mean however, that you are at a point that involves intervention. This may involve lifestyle changes, weight loss, exercise or all of the above, in most cases. That is what you are going to learn in this book, and it is all in the confines of safety. Reprinted from *Clinical Anatomy of*

the Lumbar Spine and Sacrum, 3rd Edition, Nikolai Bogduk, 211, Copyright (1997), with permission from Elsevier.

> Remember that incident I told you about, my first episode of back pain that lasted over the weekend? I did go back to jogging, occasionally lifting weights, really having no problems. Then about 3 years later, I fell with a very large male patient in the water. He couldn't break his fall, so I caught him as he fell. This time it took me 9 months to recover, and I was working full time. I simply went to bed when I got home from work each day. I slowly started back exercising, walking or doing the Nordic Trac for 5 to 10 minutes; that was all I could tolerate.

I had lost some of my spinal shock absorption through injury and aging. I was three years older, but still the same size and about the same fitness level. The spine was not quite the same, even though my physical traumas were minor; I was breaking down my back bit by bit as I pushed it, impatient and aggravated that my back was not responding to my timetable. Then, the next year, I fell again with a large male patient in the water. I did "recover" to a degree over the next year, but I was unable to go back to jogging. It finally wasn't worth the pain every time I tried to jog. "Thus, even a small lesion can substantially compromise the normal biomechanics of a disc." (Bogduk 1997, 85)

Symptoms of Degenerative Disc Disease (DDD)

With a diseased or herniated lumbar disc, there is definite loss of tolerance to increased loads on the spine. Most common are prolonged sitting, driving, repeated bending and straightening (like getting in and out of the car), and marked stiffness or pain first thing in the morning. Problems or symptoms related to disc pathology are always aggravated or intolerant to increased loading, whether it is a positional or external load, such as a heavy purse, briefcase, load of laundry, or a bag of groceries. To understand the dynamics of the disc is to understand the concept of loading. An increasing intolerance to "load" is the predominant characteristic of degenerative processes of the aging spine.

What happens now? Possibly, you don't have a herniated disc, as confirmed by an MRI. Yet, little episodes of back pain, stiffness, and loss of recovery from leisure activities are becoming more frequent. "It is known that the spine pain that precedes herniation often has a course of gradual exacerbations and remissions that somehow belie a purely mechanical explanation." (White and Panjabi 1978, 284) What is going on with your back?

Osteoarthritis of the Spine—Facet Joint Syndrome

We sustain micro-traumas to the discs from aging, job related tasks and postures, and increased collagen and loss of shock absorption in the disc. The weight bearing of additional pressures through the spine has to be taken up somewhere. These degenerative changes to the discs result in a narrowing of space in between vertebrae. The facet joints now take up the additional weight the discs are unable to bear. On an x-ray, this shows up as a diminished space between vertebrae—a thin line as opposed to greater spacing between vertebrae with a healthier disc. The two levels that wear out the quickest historically are the fourth and fifth lumbar discs. Remember the intervertebral segment is considered the disc, vertebral body and the facet joints. This is buttressed by ligamentous and muscular attachments. "With injury to the intervertebral disc the kinematics of the functional spinal unit is altered. The response of the facets to abnormal loading patterns or direct injury might be cartilage degeneration, facet atrophy, and if excessive forces are maintained over a long period, bony adaption in the form of sclerosis or spurring." (Porterfield and DeRosa 1991, 85)

Remember the facet joints allow for articulation of spinal segments upon one another. With these degenerative changes now in the articulating joints, you may notice you aren't able to turn and look over your shoulder as well when driving, bend as low for a tennis ball, or drive the golf ball quite as far. You're losing some range of motion and mobility. Hot showers help, yes, but you now get stiffer after that round of golf or tennis, or afternoon of yard work.

"It appears that increased stiffness in the intervertebral discs is the principal cause of the reduction in mobility that develops with aging." (Grelsamer and Loebl 1997, 182) There is nothing you can do to change this process; however, exercise—just moving—helps!

Movement, using your muscles, provides nutrition to the discs, joints, muscles, and ligaments—every component of the spine. But, you say it hurts to move. Ah, herein lies the beauty of water as a treatment mode. Movement in water is much less painful for many reasons, and this is discussed in detail later in the book. Now, I just want you to understand why it is important that you move.

"Cartilage nutrition is maintained by infusion and diffusion of fluids." (Calliet 1995, 203) Muscular contractions and movement of the joints and limbs, allows for the nutritional process of imbibition to occur. Imbibition is the absorption of fluid by a solid body or gel, according to Tabers Medical Dictionary.

When we stop moving, there are physiological changes in the articulating cartilage of joints. This can lead to degenerative changes that then affect the efficiency and function of the joint and disc. This is likely to happen at more than one joint in the spine. Remember the facet joints, disc and vertebrae all function as a unit. Articulation or weight bearing problems at one spinal level can lead to problems at the segment above or below, as well. With loss of range, unequal weight-bearing through the spinal segment and loss of disc shock absorption, degenerative processes set in. One of the conditions that develops with degeneration is spinal stenosis. This is a common, bothersome spinal condition that bears closer scrutiny.

Spinal Stenosis

Lumbar as well as cervical or thoracic spinal stenosis occurs when there is a loss of space within the spinal canal or foramen, the small opening where the nerve exits. Loss of this "operating space" causes a crowding on the spinal cord and nerve, causing an impingement, or what is commonly known as a pinched nerve.

What causes this loss of space? Well, in some cases, the individual was born with a smaller spinal canal. There may have been some episodes of back pain as a teenager but not too significant, most likely. When the discs begin the degenerative process and they lose height and spinal shock absorption, the vertebrae move closer together. Remember too, when the disc dynamics change, there may be the development of spurring because of changes in weight bearing. These spurs, known as osteophytes, can press on the nerve at the point where it exits the spine. These spurs may occur about the facet joints, the point of movement, or within the borders of the vertebral body itself. All of these things impose on the spinal canal and the nerves in the spine.

Another thing that imposes on this space is the herniation of the disc (HNP—herniated nucleus pulposus). A bulging of the outer annular wall or the herniation itself will encroach into the spinal canal. There are incidences where trauma or other disease processes can lead to the development of lumbar spinal stenosis. These include inflammatory diseases such as rheumatoid arthritis, infections and tumors.

Encroachment into the spinal canal can also result from fibrous ligaments that have lost elastic properties due to aging. A bulging of the disc wall will also encroach upon the spinal cord. Spinal stenosis is defined in two categories: central stenosis and lateral stenosis. Central canal stenosis occurs when there is impingement within the canal itself. Central stenosis can occur with a congenitally smaller spinal canal or when aging ligaments calcify and lose elasticity, encroaching within the central canal. Lateral stenosis occurs when there is an encroaching body on the nerve that is outside of the actual spinal cord. Lateral stenosis, also known as foraminal stenosis, presents differently than central canal stenosis.

Symptoms of Spinal Stenosis

With spinal stenosis of the lumbar spine, there is increased pain and intolerance to standing and walking. There is a feeling of weakness in one or both legs, or the sensation that the leg is going to buckle. There may be an episode(s) of falling too. Rest relieves the pain; sitting relieves the leg pain. Sitting puts the spine into flexion, a position where the vertebrae are slightly opened off of each other. This creates more space in the spinal canal, which relieves impinging pressure on the nerves. "Stenosis of the lateral canal will present with unilateral (one-sided) symptoms of buttock, thigh and even leg and foot pain." (DeFranca 1996, 124) Central spinal stenosis often presents with bilateral symptoms including achiness, numbness, weakness and parathesias into both legs.

Sciatica with spinal stenosis occurs frequently. If you have symptoms that are not relieved by any change in position, you may consider further diagnostic workup. There are other conditions that can cause chronic back pain, including abdominal aortic aneurysm (Kirkaldy-Willis). "Back pain due to degenerative disease is seldom, if ever unrelenting and usually responds to rest." (Kirkaldy-Willis 1983, 133) Another cause of chronic, extreme back pain can be cancer. Organic disease must be ruled out. Patients who have back pain along with a combination of any of the following symptoms, need further physician assessment (DeFranca 1996, 122):

- Fever and/or weight loss
- Pain at night
- Morning stiffness
- Acute, localized bone pain from fracture or bone expansion
- Visceral pain

Symptoms of lumbar spinal stenosis include intolerances to standing, walking extended distances or walking and carrying (or pushing) a load. For example, grocery shopping is the worst—tolerable only by leaning on the basket. Leaning forward opens the facets and vertebrae off each other, offering some relief. Standing in line or standing at a reception (extended standing) is murderous. If you have to be in heels during this, you're miserable by the end of the night. Many of my patients mourn the loss of their favorite past time—cooking. To spend the afternoon or evening in the kitchen preparing a dinner is a sacrifice few choose to make too often, although they'd love nothing more.

Osteoporosis

"We have heard osteoporosis referred to as an orthopedic problem, a problem resulting from hormonal imbalance, and a metabolic disorder. All are accurate."

—(Slovik 2000, 1)

Osteoporosis means porous bones. Once it was more of a mystery with its existence confirmed only with the occurrence of a fracture. It is no longer thought of as inevitable due to tremendous strides in pharmaceutical and medical research. The medical community has discovered effective steps to combat osteoporosis early on, not in mid-life or later. Diagnostic screening is available on a wide basis and has proven to be very reliable. Let's look at osteoporosis, risk factors and effective interventions.

Calcium is the most important mineral for bone formation and remodeling. Calcium is also important in the function of the heart, blood pressure, nerve and muscle tissue. We obtain calcium through the ingestion of leafy green vegetables and dairy products, and weight-bearing exercise. What you put in your body is very important. You can get calcium through supplements, but it is best to get your main source of calcium through your diet. Fruits and grains also supply calcium to lesser degrees. Vitamin D is important in the utilization of calcium; even 15 minutes a day in the sun is beneficial to getting adequate vitamin D exposure. According to the Harvard Health Publications on Osteoporosis, "calcium's protective effects are greater when consumed in the diet. Research has also indicated that dietary calcium seems to reduce the risk of high blood pressure and kidney stones. While no such effects are derived from calcium supplements." (Slovik 2000, 26)

What are the recommended values for calcium intake? The National Institutes of Health recommend "1,000 mg for premenopausal women and postmenopausal women taking estrogen; 1,200 mg for pregnant or lactating women, and 1,500 mg for postmenopausal women not on estrogen, and for all women over 65 years." (Slovik 2000, 26) Why is it so important to get calcium now? Can't I wait until I'm older? Let's look closer at that.

Osteoporosis is classified as Type I and Type II. Type I osteoporosis occurs in the perimenopausal and postmenopausal stages; this is when estrogen begins to decline. "Type I primary osteoporosis refers to the rapid loss of bone associated with estrogen decline." (Slovik 2000, 5) Bone (or calcium) loss is greatest 3 to 7 years post menopause then begins to level off. Type II primary osteoporosis is the end result of wear and tear and bone loss associated with aging; "it develops more slowly, and is usually not apparent until age 75 or older." (Slovik 2000, 5)

Our body utilizes calcium through proper nutrition, genetics, and weight-bearing exercise. As a growing child and adolescent, your activity level and nutritional habits determine the number of deposits you are making into the "calcium bank." These deposits accumulate over a period of time until you're about forty years old. "Bone mass peaks after skeletal maturity, sometime in the fourth decade." (Kaplan 1987). So, all this is well and good, but your habits and lifestyle also take out withdrawals from the bone bank, and by age 40 your withdrawals begin to outnumber your deposits—you begin to lose more calcium than you produce. "Under normal conditions (proper diet and activity), net deposits cannot be made to the bone bank after age 35." (Kaplan 1987, 8) What are some of these calcium thieves?

They are diseases such as rheumatoid arthritis, juvenile-onset diabetes, liver disease or malabsorption syndromes (like Crohn's Disease). Certain medications leach calcium from the body and these include corticosteroids, heparin and thyroid medications, all over an extended period of time.

Good habits like exercise and proper (calcium-rich) diet make deposits into the calcium bank. Bad habits—well, they rob you over a period of time. These include drinking alcohol more than 2 drinks per day; coffee—more than 3 cups a day; smoking, and a poor, highly processed diet. This diet, fast food basically, is nutrient poor by the time it finally gets to your table.

Another area of calcium theft includes malabsorption and poor estrogen production. Athletic amenorrhea—lack of a regular menstrual period from low body fat, robs calcium from the body. Anorexia and bulimia are considered a malabsorption syndrome, taking calcium away from the body (bones, tissue, heart & nerves). You can start calcium loss in your teens in these two scenarios.

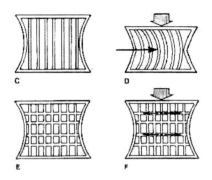

Ethnicity and gender both play a role in osteoporosis. Asians are the most likely ethnic class to have osteoporosis, followed by Caucasian women. The more petite and fair, the higher the osteoporosis risk factor. African-Americans are the least likely race to get osteoporosis, followed by the Native American Indian. Women are much more likely to get osteoporosis versus men. Men that do get this usually get the type II osteoporosis, the one associated with aging. Other possible causes for male osteoporosis include "alcoholism, use of corticosteroids, (for asthma or other inflammatory diseases) and low sex (testosterone) hormones." (Slovik *2000*, 8) See illustration C: Internal vertical struts brace the box (D). E: Transverse connections prevent the vertical struts from bowing, and increase the load-bearing capacity of the box. Reprinted from *Clinical Anatomy of the Lumbar Spine and Sacrum*, 3rd Edition, Nikolai Bogduk, 7, Copyright (1997), with permission from Elsevier.

In osteoporosis, the structural integrity of the bone is affected by the gradual loss of calcium. As the bone becomes more porous, the ability or capacity to bear weight is greatly diminished. Something as simple as lifting a box or hard coughing can result in a compression fracture in the thoracic spine, the mid-back. The internal collapse comes when the bony network, which resembles a lattice, experiences a disruption of one (or several) vertical columns or horizontal cross ties. This type of fracture may lead to stooped posture. The more stooped, the less tolerance for standing or performing of simple tasks, due to diminished capacity of the spine to bear weight. Even standing for a short duration is intolerable in the early stages of a compression fracture. This is where water exercise can be beneficial. It diminishes the amount of load (or pressure) transmitted through the spine by eliminating gravity. The buoyancy of the water is also supportive and helps diminish the pain of movement. Other less common sites for osteoporotic fractures include the hip and wrist. With hip fractures, something as simple as twisting or turning can result in a fracture or fall when osteoporosis exists. "In osteoporosis, as in hypertension, there is often a long, latent period before clinical symptoms or complications develop. The first symptoms occur when bone mass is so compromised that the skeletal framework can no longer withstand the mechanical stresses of everyday living." (Kaplan 1987, 2)

Now that we have covered the bone bank analogy, lifestyle and risk factors, we would be remiss not to mention pharmaceutical management. Huge strides have been made in research concerning osteoporosis, breast cancer and hormone replacement therapy. This debate rages on. Bone building medications such as Fosamax and Calcitonin have proven to reduce bone loss and slightly increase bone density. These are universally part of the medicinal management for osteoporosis. There are also nasal sprays with calcium. Estrogen replacement or hormonal replacement therapy (i.e. Evista) remains controversial. The complicating factor is breast cancer. This must be determined by your physician and involves several factors that will determine the course of action. This is a case by case scenario; sit down with your physician to discuss your best course of action.

The third side of the triangle, the other two being diet and medication, is exercise. Let's put exercise in the lifestyle category, along with conservative alcohol and caffeine intake and <u>no</u> smoking. You must exercise to prevent bone loss! That is weight bearing exercise. It can be as simple as walking and using hand weights. If you have a compression fracture you can start in the pool where there is a resistive environment but decreased gravity to better accommodate your pain.

"Daily weight-bearing activity is essential to the health of the skeleton. Mechanical weight bearing is perhaps the most important exogenous factor affecting bone development and remodeling." (Kaplan 1987, 13) The old adage again pops into my head: Move it or lose it. It's all about exercise—and "load." What is "load?" Keep reading. You may have to look at it several times, but it's all about to make more sense.

Other Sources of Low Back Pain

We have discussed degenerative disc disease, osteoarthritis, and spinal stenosis. There are many variations and combinations of pathology and degenerative processes that result in low back pain and loss of function. Three less common types of back pain are lumbago, spondylolisthesis and degenerative scoliosis. Lumbago is a general pain in the low back, spondylolisthesis is a forward slippage of one vertebra upon another, and degenerative scoliosis is a curvature of the spinal column as a result of degenerative changes. Let's look at each of these conditions individually.

Lumbago/Low Back Pain

Lumbago "could be used as a descriptive title for any type of back ache." (Corrigan and Matland 1993, 287) It is usually not verified by any diagnostic testing, but is sudden in onset, with severe pain and loss of spinal mobility. It usually clears up in several days with bed rest and anti-inflammatory medications, but results in a lingering, dull low back pain, even after it resolves. This may be isolated or occur fairly frequently. Causes of this back pain have been proposed as acute annular tears of the disc, movement of disc material, entrapment of cartilage within the facet joint, or even possible compression fracture related to osteoporosis. Muscle spasm and guarding accompany the sudden onset of back pain. Many times this occurs with bending over, or a bending and twisting motion. Leg pain may occur with the onset of back pain but this is not typical or of a long duration if it does occur. "In a sizeable proportion of patients the natural history of this condition does not resemble that of disc degeneration. Attacks occur periodically until they finally cease with no evidence of disc degeneration." (Corrigan and Matland 1993, 288)

Spondylolisthesis

There are several types of spondylolisthesis, which is the forward slippage of one vertebra on its lower counterpart. They include traumatic, congenital, pathological (disease-based), and degenerative, which is the classification we will discuss. The most common occurrence of spondylolisthesis is in the lower lumbar spine, at the fourth lumbar vertebrae; less common is the forward slippage of the fifth lumbar vertebrae on the sacrum. "Degenerative spondylolisthesis is four times as common in women as men and is not common below the age of 50 years." (Corrigan and Matland 1993, 251) The degree of slippage is slight to moderate and rarely indicated for surgery. The slope of the sacrum does play a part of the high predominance of spondylolisthesis at L4-5, the fourth and fifth lumbar vertebrae. Degenerative changes in the disc and at the facet joints play a role as well. Remember the facet joints hook one vertebra into the other and serve as a locking bony mechanism. "Forward slippage will not occur unless this bony hook becomes deficient." (Corrigan and Matland 1993, 250)

This forward slippage and the anatomical slope of the sacrum make standing difficult and intolerable beyond short duration. Add high heels to the equation and this further tilts the pelvis forward. With an existing spondylolisthesis, a woman attending a reception in high heels would likely have onset of low back pain within hours that might last for days. High heels here are defined as any-thing greater than 1½ inches. With a moderate spondylolisthesis, a more forward displacement of L4 on L5, there may also be episodes of sciatica. The forward slippage of the upper vertebrae on the lower vertebrae will create increased ten-sion on the exiting nerves between the fourth and fifth lumbar vertebrae.

Obviously, one would need to avoid high heels, as earlier defined. Prolonged standing should also be avoided. Strengthening of the abdominal muscles is indi-cated. A corset may lend additional abdominal compression, which is supportive of the lumbar spine. A large abdomen from excessive weight will likely aggravate an existing spondylolisthesis. Persistent sciatica and poor standing tolerance on an ongoing basis is cause for a thorough diagnostic workup by your physician.

The American Medical Association Home Medical Encyclopedia states that "lumbar spondylolisthesis is usually due to osteoarthritis in which the joints between the vertebrae become worn and unstable; thus liable to slip under stress."

Degenerative Adult Scoliosis

"Scoliosis is defined as an appreciable lateral deviation in the normally straight vertical line of the spine." (White and Panjabi 1978, 94) There are several charac-teristics of scoliosis. Most of us refer to scoliosis as a congenital (birth) condition. Scoliosis, in most cases, is detected in the pre-pubescent or adolescent teen. In other cases, such as cerebral palsy or muscular dystrophy, scoliosis can be a major concern with overall function of the cardiac or pulmonary (respiratory) systems compromised. These cases, stemming from neuromuscular diseases are most complicated and not our focus. Our focus is the development of scoliosis from other degenerative processes. Scoliosis may also evolve from trauma or surgery. In these cases, as well as other degenerative sources, there is a disruption in spinal mechanics. "Scoliosis can result from either gross or subtle disruptions of the del-icate balance." (White and Panjabi 1978, 94) This balance concerns function and symmetry between the spinal column, ligaments, and neuromuscular mechanics of all of these combined.

Somewhere along the way, something upset the balance or symmetry. That could be the symmetry between each side of the spinal column, or symmetry between the two sides of the body. This could include a leg length discrepancy, fractures, or even a previous spine surgery. Remember that the spine is comprised of seven cervical, twelve thoracic, and five lumbar vertebrae and the sacrum that operate as a congruous system. If a simple segment in the system is affected, it will effect the spine overall. Degenerative disc disease or an osteoarthritic facet can throw the system out of balance, including operating balances within the muscles and ligaments, as well as the articulating spine.

There are two types of adult scoliosis: idiopathic which means we don't know what caused it, and degenerative scoliosis. Degenerative scoliosis results secondary to other degenerative changes in the spine.

In adult idiopathic scoliosis, the scoliosis most likely was present in adolescence and simply went unnoticed or untreated. With idiopathic scoliosis there may be a very gradual progression of the scoliotic curve, about one-degree annually. It hasn't been symptomatic for years, but the very gradual progression of the curve with time and degenerative changes has suddenly (it seems) made this minor scoliosis very painful and problematic. That curve has progressed significantly. Fortunately, the degenerative arthritic changes in the spine eventually arrests further scoliotic changes. Actually, the stiffening of the spine with arthritic changes also lends stability. Adult idiopathic scoliosis usually has a thoracic (upper back) curve, predominately to the right.

The second type of scoliosis is degenerative and is a result of osteoarthritic changes of the spine. This type of scoliosis primarily appears later in life in the lumbar spine. Remember, more weight bearing and mobility occurs in the lumbar spine, especially at the 4th and 5th vertebrae. This accounts for the higher degenerative changes in the lower spine. Surprisingly, there is a much higher incidence of scoliosis in women, about 4:1 ratio. Some thoughts are that this has a hormonal basis.

Back Principles and Treatment

Once you have suffered a significant back injury, your life will change. "Significant" means you suffered some disability over a period of time—greater than five months. You may have lost time at work, lost your job, had to change jobs, had to give up some leisure activities, or had some alteration in the family dynamics secondary to the physical pain and dysfunction from your injury. You may even have undergone surgery.

What now? You aren't the person you once were, nor will you ever be. However, your life is not over! There will still be activities to enjoy, maybe the same ones, but with some modification. You will need to adopt some level of exercise as part of your lifestyle now in order not to be victimized by back pain. How much exercise and what you can do safely and comfortably will need to be determined by you, your doctor, and a qualified therapist, be that physical or occupational therapist, athletic trainer or some combination of the above. I highly recommend doing some type of rehab initially so you can learn what you can do safely in reference to your particular type of back problem. Remember that back pain is gray. As varied as the sources, or combined sources of back pain can be, there is a common weave in all of this.

Every single person with back pain goes through the processes of (1) loading; (2) creep, and (3) "optimal loading zone," (Porterfield and DeRosa 1991, 13) which I refer to as "the window of tolerance." When you understand these three principles, you have the tools for effective pain management.

The purpose of this book is educating you about the anatomy of the spine, degenerative changes and making smarter choices. You can make smarter choices when you learn specifically about loading, creep, and the window of tolerance. By learning about your type of back problem and working with a qualified therapist, you can develop a new point of reference, choose your tasks and leisure activities appropriately, and better plan your day. Let's look in depth at load, creep, and window of tolerance—all critical to understanding your back pain.

LOADING

The 2001 *Webster's Unabridged Dictionary of English Language* has 39 definitions for the word "load." The fourth and fifth definition are: "(4) the quantity borne or sustained by something," and "(5) the weight supported by a structure or part."

A load bearing structure can refer to the disc, ligament, or joint. Certain postures or tasks increase the force applied to this structure, whether a joint or disc.

A motion or posture that heavily loads the disc and facet joint is rotation. Rotation combined with bending and twisting is the most erosive motion to the spine over a period of time. Don't you recall many professional golfers and tennis players that have suffered from back pain? Now you know why. "Clinical evidence of annular disruption implies that the disc has failed due to some combination of bending, torsion and tension." (White and Panjabi 1978, 9)

There are two types of load: dynamic and static. Dynamic load is a compressive force that occurs in addition to movement. Static load is a compressive load that is sustained over a period of time and involves no or negligible motion.

Dynamic Loading

When you are standing, you are 100% weight-bearing. Climbing stairs increases the load over 100% because you are using force to lift and move the entire body upstairs, or up an incline. The increase in pressure, or load, is borne through the discs, cartilage, tendons and ligaments. Another example of dynamic loading is grocery shopping. You push the grocery cart, and as you fill it up, the load becomes greater and more and more effort is required to move it. For an injured back, this additional weight quickly overloads the spine. Back pain in the form of spasms or sciatica may occur within hour(s) of your trip to the grocery store.

How about carrying a toddler or pet? What about walking a medium to large-sized dog and counteracting the load he produces when he strains on the leash? This is dynamic loading. Wait until he sees a squirrel or cat and really jerks against the leash.

Mowing the yard is dynamically loading the spine. You have to push the mower hard enough to overcome the resistance of the grass. If the grass is wet or fairly high, then that much more effort is required. A self-propelled mower makes a world of difference here I've found out; it is worth the money. Dragging a long water hose through the yard—additional loading of the spine. All of these common everyday tasks are so simple. Yet, they can quickly make an injured or weak back very angry. There are many more examples of dynamic loading; these are just a few to get you thinking.

The back is working all the time. We take it for granted because we do so much automatically. You don't have to do something that is obviously dangerous such as carrying a 50lb. bag of fertilizer, or carrying or pulling a heavy bag when travelling. Let's look at another type of loading that is so insidious, it really leaves you clueless.

Static Loading

A. L. Nachemson, the renowned researcher, physician and author, did a breakthrough study (Nachemson 1976, 59) that measured disc pressure of the third lumbar disc (L3) according to different postures and tasks. Reference the illustration. You'll see in standing that there is 100 kilograms of force (kg/f) translating through the lumbar spine, specifically L3. Sitting is 140 kg/f (more pressure on the disc than in standing). Straight leg raises increases the L3 disc pressure to 150 kg/f. What about ab crunches—aren't those supposed to be good for back problems? You see that they increase the pressure in the L3 to 210 kg/f! This is equivalent to lifting 44 lbs. with a straight back! Brushing your teeth or shaving produces 120 kg/f.

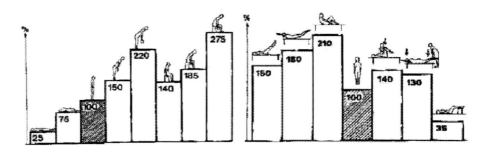

Figure courtesy of Nachemson, A.L.: *The lumbar spine: an orthopedic challenge.* Spine, 1:59, 1976.

You get the idea. The back never gets a break; everyday activities are stressing the lumbar spine. Some of these are static postures. Dynamic loading produces much greater pressures. The back needs some help! Strengthening the trunk, among other things, really helps offset some of this constant loading. One note of interest before we move on. You know how sometimes lying on the floor (or bed) and just getting your knees up seems to relieve back pain and spasms? You see in the illustration that this particular posture reduces the load to 35 kilograms of force! That makes sense now. You understand that loading really does make a difference. Let's move on to the real culprit, now that you understand dynamic and static loading.

CREEP

No, this isn't the bully from school who used to make you miserable, although creep can make you feel pretty bad! "Creep is the deformation that follows the initial loading of a material and occurs as a function of time." (White and Panjabi 1978, 98) Simply, creep is a process that occurs after a material (tissue, ligaments, muscle or discs) takes on additional pressure that results in a deformation, or change, as time goes on. The longer you sustain a certain posture, such as sitting and working at the computer, then a deforming change occurs in the material (tissue). Creep is a "time-dependent phenomena associated with biological tissues." (Whiting and Zernicke 1998, 77) Over a period of time, with a sustained or static load, the resistance or load capacity of the tissue is reached and then deformation begins. What are we talking about here? Minutes, hours or what? Think about sustained postures that involve time. Creep is going to occur when sitting in the movies, at dinner, or riding in the car. I have had lots of patients come in with a flare-up of back pain after a long car trip. They simply wouldn't break up the trip, which would have broken up the creep process.

Tissue has a physiological range of load or pressure that it can safely and effectively sustain. Injury occurs when a load exceeds tissue tolerance. This might occur in a high-load sudden impact, such as a fall or motor vehicle accident. However, we are looking at a physiological tissue range that is overwhelmed as a function of time—a sustained posture. We are talking about a 90-minute window.

Studies by Kazarian found creep to occur over a duration of 90 minutes after which time it plateaued. (Kazarian 1975, 3-18) That is within a duration of 90 minutes, not starting at 90 minutes. In fact, creep can start within 20 minutes, but it affects each person differently. You may go to dinner with friends and find yourself shifting this way and that while others can seemingly sit at will for long periods of time. Unfortunately, your disc is probably in worse degenerative shape than is theirs. "The non-degenerated discs creep slowly and reach their final deformation after considerable time, as compared to degenerated discs." (White and Panjabi 1978, 9) As we know, degenerative discs lose a degree(s) of shock-absorbing capacities and the ability to uniformly distribute load. Discs experience creep as well as ligaments and bone. Just as creep can occur in the low back over the duration of a sustained posture, so can an injured or arthritic knee experience that same dull ache and stiffness after prolonged sitting. Creep is a function of time. "Creep deformation is greater and occurs more rapidly in the injured joint, which tends to creep in the direction of injury." (Kirkaldy-Willis 1983, 26)

There are factors that affect the onset of creep. These are discussed in depth by Whiting and Zernicke in the <u>Biomechanics of Musculoskeletal Injury</u>, Human Kinetics Publishing, 118–121. Let's look at some factors influencing load and creep.

<u>Age</u>. As we age, our tissue loses some of its resistance, strength and density. Injury occurs more often and recovery takes longer. "It is important to recognize, however, the difference between chronological age and physiological age." (Whiting and Zernicke 1998, 118) The quality of tissue could be younger physiologically versus actual chronological age due to fitness level and healthy habits. Conversely, poorer tissue health would result from previous injury, smoking, or lifestyle.

<u>Gender</u>. This will be influenced by hormones, muscle mass and activity levels.

<u>Physical Condition</u>. Level of fitness, activity level, lifestyle habits, weight.

<u>Nutrition</u>. You are what you eat, or don't eat. "Diet provides the raw materials to build, sustain, and repair the body's tissues and therefore plays an indirect yet essential role in injury biomechanics." (Whiting and Zernicke 1998, 118)

<u>Psychological State</u>. Stress, depression and coping mechanisms greatly impact the level of back pain and recovery.

<u>Fatigue</u>. "Physical and mental fatigue increase the likelihood of injury because of compromised muscle strength, coordination, mental attentiveness and concentration." (Whiting and Zernicke 1998, 119)

<u>Previous Injury</u>. Areas of previous injury will not have the same tissue resistance or loading capacity.

<u>Disease</u>. This could include rheumatoid arthritis, Paget's Disease or diabetes, to name a few.

<u>Body Type</u>. Size plays a role in injury predisposition and recovery. This includes height, weight, muscle mass versus fatty tissue, and body type.

<u>Inflammation/Pain</u>. "Tissue that is acutely inflamed will have significantly reduced tissue loading tolerance with a much faster onset of pain. With the onset of pain, activity avoidance takes place as a means of pain management." (Whiting and Zernicke 1998, 120)

<u>Bone Integrity</u>. "Any disease or injury that compromises (bone) performance jeopardizes the structural integrity of both the affected bone and the skeletal system in general."(Whiting and Zernicke 1998, 122)

I want you to be an educated consumer. This is your body, your back, and it has to last a lifetime. When you have an awareness of factors that affect your back, positively or negatively, you can make smarter choices. There are many things you can do to make positive inroads in the management of your back pain.

You don't have to be a prisoner to your back. However, you must participate in the care and management of your pain. You may need some intervention along the way in the form of physical therapy or chiropractic, or even injections or surgery, but at some point, it becomes your responsibility.

THE WINDOW PRINCIPLE

I often tell my patients there is a "window of tolerance" within which their recovery (which includes rehabilitation exercises) occurs. It is the job of the therapist and patient to identify the parameters of this window. In other words, you want to exercise enough to promote healing in the form of gained strength and endurance. However, there's a high end to the "window," when too much activity, or a specific activity, will overload the tissue and actually exacerbate the tissue. This results in a flare-up of symptoms. "Tissues of the musculoskeletal system have a common denominator: they all require the stimulus of nondestructive stresses to maintain their health." (Porterfield and DeRosa 1991, 12)

Nondestructive stresses are stresses applied within the window of tissue tolerance—enough to stimulate growth but non enough to break down tissue by overloading it. Tissue breakdown can occur as much by over-training as a sedentary lifestyle.

There are three main areas that define this "optimal loading zone" or window of tolerance. These are age, adaptive changes and injury.

(1) Age. With aging, we lose the hydrating and elastic properties of musculoskeletal and bony tissue. With this comes an increased fibrosis of the tissue which accounts for the increased overall stiffness and longer recovery time from injury that we experience. With aging, we are no longer able to "withstand the magnitude and duration of forces" we formerly tolerated. Don't tell me what you did two, three, or five years ago, because it is no longer relevant. It is different now because 1) you are older, and 2) you have sustained an injury that is going to alter the tissue loading tolerance. I didn't say you couldn't or wouldn't get better, but it will be nearly impossible to recover 100% of your pre-injury state.

(2) Adaptive Changes. Most of us have gotten less active as we have gotten older. Family obligations, job obligations, physical changes (such as weight gain) have led to decreased activity. With the rise of technology, we spend more and more time in front of our computers, DVDs, VCRs and TVs. Unfortunately, our children are doing the same. With the rise in sedentary lifestyle, for whatever reasons, comes "adaptive changes in the form of connective tissue shortening and

muscle weakness" (Porterfield and DeRosa 1991, 14) and decreased tolerance to stresses on the musculoskeletal system. We can't do as much! We have lost some of our physical capacities in the form of strength, endurance, flexibility and coordination.

(3) Injury. We heal from injuries, but the repaired tissue will not have the former loading capacity we had prior to injury. "The end result is repair with a tissue related in structure but different from the original tissue that was damaged. There is, in effect a new and now lowered maximal limit of tissue tolerance." (Porterfield and DeRosa 1991, 14-15) You must exercise to maintain, or recover, the health of your musculoskeletal tissue, but this must happen within the window of tolerance.

The optimal loading zone isn't comprised only of rehabilitative exercises. Activities of daily living must be figured into this window, too. This is where many people get into trouble. Let's review some activities of daily living that cause an increased load on the lumbar spine. Refer back to the study by Dr. Nachemson in the discussion of "load," and how different postures increase or decrease pressure in the lumbar spine.

As you recover from an episode of back pain, eventually you will start exercising. I gage my patients' recovery initially by how well they are handling everyday activities. They first have to tolerate daily life without an increase in symptoms before I really start in with a dedicated rehab exercise program. If my patient cannot tolerate driving carpool, how can they be ready for exercises beyond this level of loading? Your window of tolerance will change as you heal, but you must be patient and respect this stage of recovery.

When I hurt my back the second time, my sitting tolerance dropped to practically nothing. I could sit at the most for 10 minutes and I was working full time! So, I didn't sit to do my paperwork; I stood. My tolerance for standing was greater than my sitting tolerance.

Remember the study by Dr. Nachemson on the different postures and their generated load on the spine? Standing is 100 kg/f through the lumbar spine while sitting is slightly higher. Sitting and leaning slightly forward is 120 kg/f. These postures are common when working on the computer, or sitting in the bleachers at our children's ballgames. Standing generated less load on my spine than sitting. I know executives who have placed drafting tables at their workplace because they better tolerate standing, or can alternate between standing and sitting. Making the bed, vacuuming, or mopping are all activities that aggravate back pain in many people. Walking the dog increases load on the spine because you have to pull back enough on the leash that you overcome the force of the dog's body weight and his exertion as he strains on the leash. Depending on the state of your back, even a small dog can produce more load than your back is able to tolerate at that point. Ouch!

My point is this—you must respect the back's window of tolerance. Initially, this window will only be activities of daily life. As you get stronger, this window will change, but it won't happen overnight. Getting impatient and pushing it, may likely lead to a flare-up. Figure daily tasks within the window of tolerance. If you are going to your child's ballgame that night, don't try to clean the entire house; or, don't sit all day at the computer and then go to dinner or a movie that night without expecting to pay for it the next day. If you cannot avoid a day like this every now and then, try to make the next day a little more forgiving; don't pack it full of activities. Remember loading the spine isn't solely about exercise—consider activities of daily life.

Remember earlier how we talked about musculoskeletal weakness could come from disease or overuse? Defining your window of loading tolerance will have you doing a level of exercise that stimulates endurance and strength building but not to the point that tissue tolerance is overwhelmed and flare-up occurs. When you eventually define this window, respect it. There is a cut off point with exercising.

Let's look at two examples of overuse. Ann was a triathlete. She worked out all the time, at all hours, and worked out everyday. It seems like she would be really strong working this much, right? I don't know about that. She was plagued by chronic nagging injuries—a pulled muscle here, low back pain one day, sciatica the next, tendonitis at different joints. All of this was fairly constant but only occasionally bad enough to "make" her have to take a day off. She really wasn't as strong as someone doing a similar program just 3-4 days a week. By not allowing for recovery from constant loading of the joints, she was actually breaking down tissue. She was doing this consistently enough that she was actually shrinking her window of tolerance. Respect your body and allow it to heal itself. It is self-defeating to rush the process. Remember, the back is "king;" it will always win in this type of show down.

The second example is Joe, a 63-year old accountant, and an avid runner dealing with some nagging sciatica. He couldn't run his usual 10 miles per day; in fact, he could barely run four miles, but he kept trying, regardless. He learned about loading tolerance and seemed to understand. He did, he just couldn't accept it. He finally worked up to jogging 4-6 miles, 3 to 4 days a week without pain. Then he took a trip. He just couldn't contain himself: 10 miles jogging barefoot on the beach. His three months of recovery were wiped out just like that. He was back at square one, now with chronic sciatica. It took four more months to get back to tolerating 3-4 mile jogs, 3 to 4 days a week. By overdoing it and pushing his body beyond what he knew was his level of tolerance, he set himself back four months, and narrowed his window of tolerance by injuring the tissue. My analogy is this—if you bang your head against the wall once—it hurts. Do it again and again and again, and it still hurts every time! Respect the process and learn to be happy with your window of loading tolerance. It saves a lot of grief down the road.

The Value of Exercise

WHY EXERCISE?

By Howard Cotler, M.D.

Exercise is important to everyone. The coach says, "use it or lose it." The doctor says, "physical inactivity leads to the deterioration of many body functions." The employer says, "work or go home, but don't take drugs on the job site." They physical therapist says, "no pain, no gain." People/patients says, "I go to work everyday, when I get home I am exhausted and I am really not an exercise person." All of these comments create confusion, anxiety and concern. It really does not have to be a big deal—just do it. Exercise can be fast, simple and effectively incorporated into your daily life. One can climb stairs instead of taking the elevator, park at the far end of the parking lot, stretch when waiting, exercise during part of the lunch hour or just walk around the block. Do something.

So much pain and so many diseases are preventable with exercise. Prevention is easier than treatment. It is easier to start now at square one rather than come to the doctor and have to work very hard just to get "back to" square one. There is a choice and it is your choice.

Pain is the symptom that brings the majority of patients into the medical system. The Hippocratic Oath instructs physicians to attempt to limit the suffering of the human condition. Voltaire once wrote that the purpose of the physician in treating back pain was to amuse the patient while nature cured the disease. Newer forms of treatment for various musculoskeletal maladies have taken the sport medicine approach where restoration of function rather than, or in addition, to the alleviation of pain has become a treatment goal. Yet, it should be noted that both the goals of restoration of function and pain relief can coexist.

The "disuse syndrome" as advanced by Bortz (Bortz 1984, 1) has proposed the idea that our culture has become sedentary and thus has created the "human ill-being." Thus physical inactivity leads to a deterioration of many body functions, which include:

- Cardiovascular (e.g. heart disease, hypertension)
- Musculoskeletal (e.g. osteoporosis, lack of strength)
- Obesity (e.g. diabetes)
- Mental (e.g. depression, loss of self esteem, lack of energy)
- Cancer
- Accelerated aging

Inactivity and disuse can be modeled in both humans and experimental animals through immobilization. Enforced bed rest causes a loss of protein per day that originates from muscle breakdown (catabolism). Thus, disuse leads to atrophy of specific organ systems (such as the cardiovascular and/or musculoskeletal systems) and overall decline of body functions. With disuse, muscles get smaller and lose mass and ultimately lose strength. This results in a weakening of all muscle fibers in the body—arms, legs, back, heart, blood vessels, intestines, etc. Healing tissue which is immobilized tends to produce nonfunctional scar tissue with low strength. "Since some type of connective tissue exists almost everywhere in the body, the effects of aging superimposed on inactivity are widespread." (Lewis and Bottomley 1994, 263)

With an acute injury, the initial phase of tissue repair (24–48 hours) requires decreased activity to allow for healing. Bed rest, decreased movement of an injured part and pain relief are needed. During recovery the next 3 to 42 days of healing will continue to consolidate and heal if supported by maintenance of strength and flexibility exercise. With increased physical activity, peripheral and central nervous system catecholamine content is increased. This phenomenon often results in less required pain medications and thus may account for the body's own production of pain killers or beta-endorphins. These neurohumoral agents are reported to be very potent endogenous analgesics, often having 20 times the potency of exogenously administered. Less narcotics, alcohol, and tobaccos will result in better sleep patterns, which promotes healing.

The American College of Sports Medicine (ACSM 1990) has recommended an exercise program for healthy adults. Their recommendations include the following:

- Frequency—3 to 5 days per week

- Intensity—60% to 90% maximum heart rate or 50% to 80% maximum oxygen intake

- Duration—20 to 60 minutes continuous aerobic activity

- Mode—large muscle group

- Resistance training—8 to 12 repetitions of 8 to 10 exercises twice per week

Additionally, the American College of Sports Medicine in (ACSM 1978) recommended those workers whose jobs were considered physically demanding, i.e. material handlers, nurses and truck drivers, should be involved in an exercise program 3 to 5 times per week, for 30 to 40 minutes to be appropriately prepared to work. The positive effect of exercise is the observation that it affords the change to a healthier lifestyle. Those who exercise tend to take better care of themselves by decreasing or stopping tobacco, alcohol and/or drugs, eat healthier foods and tend to be thinner. It has been shown that weak muscles are a contributing factor to low back injuries and subsequently low back pain. Yet, strength and endurance training can prevent low back injuries.

In summary, we exercise for health. "Life is movement, movement is life." (American College of Sports Medicine 1978) When you are young, you exercise to strengthen your body and your mind. As one ages, there is a gradual loss of abilities. A regular exercise program can delay the aging process and allow one to live a fully active and productive life. With injury, function rather than pain relief is the main goal. Pain is likely to diminish or resolve as function increases. If this is not the case, then further diagnostic studies are warranted. We should all make exercise a part of our daily life.

WHY EXERCISE?—STAGES OF RECOVERY

"Muscular disuse leads to weakness, incoordination, atrophy and loss of flexibility."

—(Liebenson 1996, 13)

The function of the body is interconnected. The old song, "the ankle bone is connected to the knee bone, the knee bone to the hip bone" and so on has a lot of truth to it literally and figuratively. Recovering from injury, disuse, or surgery is a step-by-step process if you want long term results. You work not only on site specific strengthening, but overall endurance, coordination, and strengthening of surrounding structures. The four components of a good rehabilitation program focus on flexibility, endurance, strength and coordination—in that order. Each area builds on the previous one. Let's look more closely at each area. "Exercise training has positive effects on bone, muscle and associated connective tissue; the entire musculoskeletal system undergoes a coordinated adaptation." (Baechle and Earle 1994, 71)

Flexibility

You never want to strengthen muscles until they have achieved their full functional range of motion. Once you achieve full functional range or flexibility around an injury, then the strengthening of surrounding muscle groups will be more balanced and lead to more joint stability. Loss of flexibility, a natural occurrence of aging, plays a significant role in injuries or falls. Tissue, ligaments, tendons and fascia lose their extensibility as they become more collagenous with aging. "It is not clear whether this decreased flexibility occurs as a consequence of biological aging, degenerative disease, inactivity or some combination of these factors. (ACSM 1998, 504)

In the ACSM Resource Manual, Denise Fredette, M.S., P.T., covers several key points in her chapter on flexibility. "Avoid aggressive stretching of tissues that have been immobilized. Tissues become dehydrated and lose tensile strength during immobilization." (Fredette 1998, 457) You can't start off like gang busters with recovering tissue or tissue that is unaccustomed to tension and load. Allow the tissue to accommodate to the new demands of load and tension and do not force it. Mild soreness may occur initially, but should resolve within 24 hours. "Do not over-stretch weak muscles. Combine strengthening and stretching exercises so that gains in mobility coincide with gains in strength and stability." (Fredette 1998, 457) Gains in strength and flexibility are possible with appropriate exercising, regardless of one's age.

Endurance

Webster's New World Roget's Thesaurus defines endurance as "fortitude, stamina, capacity to endure." Oxford Pocket American Dictionary (2002) defines it as "the ability to withstand prolonged strain." Guess what? Prolonged strain IS daily life, especially with low back pain. It could include grocery shopping, attending a reception, teaching, driving carpool, tending to small children, walking a large dog, or making a bed. All of these tasks of daily life require a sustained amount of tissue tolerance and tissue loading. Everyone falls at a different place along this continuum of tissue tolerance.

Working in the water is easier due to the negligible forces of gravity. It seems so easy, yet you are working against a constant resistance—water. Patients are surprised when they are sore from what is perceived as so little. "Muscle endurance is increased by training against a resistance that can be repeated many times." (Whiting and Zernicke 1998, 110)

The more you can endure, the more you will increase the size of the window of tolerance and your tissue loading capacity. The gains in endurance translate into a greater supply of muscle energy.

Strength

With gains in flexibility and a good foundation of endurance, one can now focus on strengthening. Joint stability is improved through strengthening. There are gains in ligament strength and stiffness which further enhance the stability of a degenerative joint. Loss of joint and tissue integrity can be a result of injury related trauma, surgery or a degenerative process or disease. Without these things, we lose strength.

"Maximal strength in men and women is generally reached between the ages of 20-30 years. The strength level tends to plateau through the age of 50, followed by a decline in strength that accelerates by 65 years of age and beyond." (Whiting and Zernicke 1998, 109) With losses of strength occurring through aging or injury, there must be some intervention to arrest and prevent joint instability as much as possible. Water accommodates joint or tissue loading intolerance because of negligible gravity. There are not the compressive loads on joints and tissue in the water as there are on land. You can cut compressive loads anywhere from 50% to 100% of body weight in the water. If one cannot tolerate exercise on land then do strengthening exercises in the water. "Stronger muscles absorb more of the attendant stress on a joint, thereby reducing stress placed on affected joint surfaces." (Fredette 1998, 452)

Coordination

We have discussed flexibility, endurance and strength and now have the concluding stage of rehabilitation—coordination. By progressively working through the previous stages of flexibility, endurance and strength, one is now at the point of exercising aggressively in multiple planes without fear of injury—exercising in 3-D, in essence.

In daily life as well as in leisure activities, you move through multiple planes of range of motion with bending, twisting, leaning to side, or reaching forward or to the side. Getting in and out of the car can become burdensome and challenging with a back problem. Going from sitting to standing is a feat as well, and sometimes this one doesn't get much easier.

To move fluidly through multiple planes of range, one has to have progressed sequentially through the rehabilitation phases of flexibility, endurance and strengthening. Deconditioning affects each of these areas which in turn affects overall joint stability. Without these components in place, the systems involved in balance and coordination of movement are soon affected. "Balance is impaired after both acute and chronic inactivity. Prolonged reaction times are associated with chronic inactivity." (Lewis and Bottomley 1994, 256)

If you want any consistent relief from back pain, you must think. Learn through trial and error what is going to work for you. Different things work for each person. You can get to a much better place with your back through consistency and commitment. Let's look now at a program I have successfully used over the years to address flexibility, endurance, strengthening and coordination.

Therapeutic Water Exercises for Back Pain

"Water therapy is an excellent method to use when normal gravity conditions might make the rehabilitation process difficult, painful and even dangerous."

—(Winston 1995, vii)

THERAPEUTIC PROPERTIES OF WATER

The argument for exercise has been effectively made. The benefits are evident physically and mentally on many levels. It is imperative in recovery from injury or surgery as Dr. Cotler pointed out in his chapter on exercise, "healing tissue which is immobilized tends to produce nonfunctional scar tissue with low strength." He also reported that the first 3 to 42 days of healing continue "if supported by maintenance and flexibility exercise." Many of you are nodding your head in agreement, flashing back on how you were rooted out of bed the day after a surgery; now you understand why.

So, we've made the argument for exercise. You say, "I would give anything to exercise, but it hurts so much to move, I simply cannot." Let's qualify that statement a bit. It hurts to move on LAND when there is 100% weight bearing, compressive load on your joints or spine. As we know too, those joints and surrounding tissue may be altered by previous injury, arthritic changes, scar tissue or advancing age. There may have also been loss of flexibility, range of motion or increased loads through weight gain or injury. Clearly, intervention is needed to prevent further complications. It is not a lost cause; almost everyone can exercise in water. Here is your intervention, your starting point.

Water has been described as the perfect therapeutic medium. It has little to no compressive force (gravity). The deeper you go in the water the less gravity you battle. This allows for greater ease of movement.

When you can move more freely, you can address areas of limitation such as loss of flexibility and joint range of motion. "Move it or lose it" definitely applies to joint range of motion. With the alleviation of gravity, one can move the body, take the arms, legs and hips through their full functional range, and stretch the surrounding muscles, ligaments and tendons at the same time. By moving, you prevent loss of range in your joints and stimulate your muscles by stretching them to their greatest potential length. Movement keeps everything functioning biomechanically. This allows you to move better in day to day activities that may now be challenging—such as turning over in bed, getting out of bed in the morning, getting in and out of the car and up and down from a low chair, reaching up into a cabinet or closet, or bending over to pick up even the lightest of objects. These are things one took for granted before dealing with a back injury. Move it or lose it.

People think they aren't doing much when they work in the water because it is much easier to move; believe it or not, you can overdo it in the water. Water is deceiving in this way. You are moving more freely yes, but you are stretching tissue and moving joints into a range they are unaccustomed to on a daily basis. You will get sore. Also, you are working against the resistance of the water. It doesn't seem like much because the usual limiting force, gravity, has been eliminated and it functioned as a feedback loop for you.

By working against resistance you build endurance. As you begin to build endurance you develop a base, or foundation, upon which you can further build. This is how you expand your window of loading tolerance. It is critical that you develop a base from which to build or you will fall into a cycle of re-injury.

Finally, "by working in a multidirectional resistive environment, better overall strength in the body or specific body part can be developed." (White 1995, 6) In the water, one can effectively work opposing muscle groups to better develop muscle symmetry. If each muscle group around a joint is equally worked and developed, this helps stabilize that area or joint. Muscles help stabilize an area that may be otherwise limited by arthritic changes, structural deficits, or scar tissue. Work to develop opposing muscle groups to buttress an injured joint or area of deficit. Let's look at an example.

Sam had a total hip replacement 8 years ago on his right hip. He did fairly well after the surgery but really let himself fall into inactivity since then, even gaining 20 extra pounds of fat. Now he is feeling the effects of degenerative disc disease, early morning stiffness, stiffness with prolonged sitting and driving, and decreased endurance from weight gain and inactivity. He is starting to have right buttock pain on a frequent basis, too.

He is going in the water to exercise and to unload those degenerating spinal joints, hip joints and degenerating discs. He can now move better so he can move more, reclaiming some lost joint range of motion and muscle flexibility. By moving more, he is going to gain strength and overall endurance. By gaining strength in those postural muscles of the back, he is going to offset some of his low back pain.

By moving his right hip in different directions (forward, backward, in and out), he is going to develop better muscle symmetry around that right hip joint. As the muscle development between opposing muscle groups occurs, joint stabilization of that right hip will occur as well. After all of this happens, right buttock pain should greatly dissipate and his low back pain will disappear as trunk strength and stability improve.

With gains in all these areas we hope Sam commits himself to exercise as a lifestyle to prevent future spine and joint problems, and simply enjoy a nicer existence. I am now going to show you a comprehensive group of water exercises that will lead you out of injury or disability and into a more functional and harmonious existence with your back.

THERAPEUTIC PROPERTIES OF WATER

The most obvious benefit of getting in the water is the virtual elimination of gravity. We are talking about load, right? That is the limiting factor of many people in conventional rehabilitation—intolerance to "land" exercise due to altered tolerance to loading. That could include a person with a herniated disc, an arthritic knee, a stenotic lumbar spine or someone with osteoporosis. Yet these individuals are in dire need of exercise. Many times, these persons drop out of physical therapy after a short times because rehab is so painful. Granted, it is never fun, but these individuals didn't get the payoff of progress while enduring the pain. The answer is water therapy.

The virtual elimination of compressive forces enables one to start into the stages of recovery that include regaining flexibility, endurance, strength and coordination. The water provides a safer and more comfortable medium to work on rehabilitation. "Weakness, joint or limb swelling, loss of motion or flexibility, and overall loss of endurance are safely addressed in the aquatic environment." (White 1995, 5) Doctors are not hesitant to put a post-operative back patient in the water three to four weeks after surgery because of safety. That also includes someone with sciatica, a joint replacement or arthritic spine.

In water, one can graduate the weight-bearing. Chest-high water eliminates approximately 70% of the body weight. In waist-high water, one is about 50% weight bearing; you eliminate half of your body weight and the compressive loads on the spine and other joints. Arthritic joints require strengthening to gain stability. An arthritic or stenotic spine will experience tremendous pain relief in deep water. In deep water one is 100% non-weight bearing and arthritic joints can be distracted off of one another.

Certain conditions may preclude participation in water exercise or at least require medical clearance. These include any of the following (White 1995, 4):

- Open wounds
- Infectious skin conditions
- Severe hypertension or hypotension
- Allergies to pool chemicals
- Seizures
- Diminished respiratory capacity
- Surgical sutures
- Bladder or vaginal infections.

I would like to add dementia, incontinence, and vertigo to this list.

WATER EXERCISE PROGRAM FOR SPINE CONDITIONS

The program presented in the following pages is a basic trunk stabilization training with a focus on flexibility. Each exercise is outlined in the technique paragraph, followed by suggested repetitions and any special concerns or adaptations specific to that exercise.

It is in a format that is sequential, starting with a warm-up, then lower extremity stretching before moving into the resistive trunk strengthening and stability exercises. As noted in several exercises, there may be discomfort in performing the exercises. Avoid it if that is the case.

Ideally, it is best to discuss this program with your doctor, physical or occupational therapist, or licensed athletic trainer. This is in no way a substitution for medical advice. Talk to someone familiar with your type of back pain or any other medical condition. Good luck with your program. Remember, with back pain, moderation is the key.

ILLUSTRATED EXERCISES

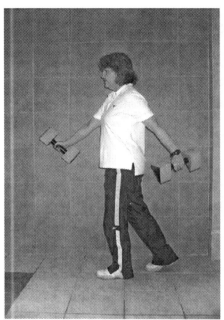 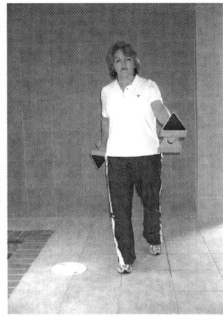

Forward Walks

Technique: Walk forward in chest high water. Swinging your arms will bring in more trunk muscles, working on trunk stabilizers and spinal mobility. Be sure you use an exaggerated walk to ensure opposite arm to opposite leg motion. Repetition: 5 laps to 5 minutes. Adaptation: One can use barbells to add more resistance to the exercise and better work trunk rotators and trunk stabilizing muscles.

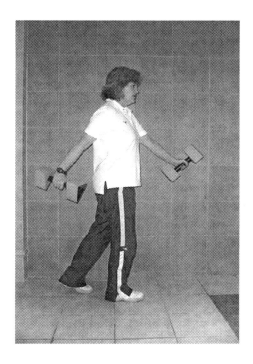

Backward Walking

Technique: Walk backwards in pool by keeping the knees locked and leg stiff, almost dragging it as you reach backward. Reach back with the toes and maintain contact with the pool floor at all times. Do not bend the knees or pick the leg up and down. It doesn't really matter where your arms are in this exercise, they are for balance assistance only. Don't use them too much for assistance, use your back and legs to move through the water. Repetition: At least 5 laps and up to 5 minutes, continuously if possible. Adaptation: If you have spinal stenosis or acute sciatica, this exercise may actually increase your pain. If this is the case, avoid this exercise.

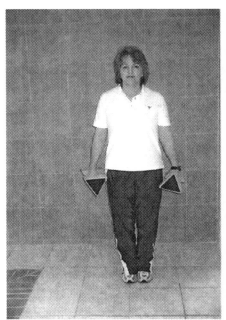 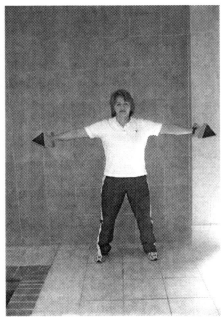

Sidestepping

Technique: This exercise works the inner and outer thighs, hips and lower back. It isolates each side to work on one-sided weakness or inflexibility, whichever is the case. Keep your feet pointing straight ahead and do not allow them to turn out. Lead with the side of your foot, not your toes. Do not turn around on this exercise when you reach the other side of the pool. Face the same direction at all times, leading with one side/leg going across, and the opposite leg when coming back. Repetition: Anywhere from 5 laps to 5 minutes, whatever is tolerable. Adaptation: You can use small barbells with this exercise. Arms and legs open as you step out, then pull them down to your sides as you step together. Arms open, legs open, legs together, arms together. You can use arms only with this exercise, too, or add the barbells.

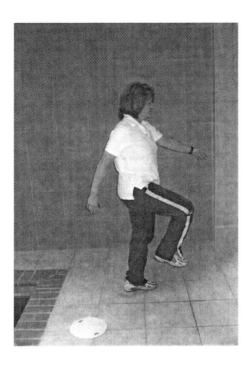

Marching

Technique: Marching works on hip range of motion, balance, and low back flexibility. This can be done in place, if necessary, but it is best to do marching across the pool so you work on dynamic balance. Arms are used for balance only. Repetition: Five laps to 5 minutes, whatever is tolerable. If you have arthritic knees, this exercise may be uncomfortable. Do what you can tolerate if your knees are a problem. Adaptation: You may march in place if needed. Raise knees to tolerable height, preferably 45 to 90 degrees.

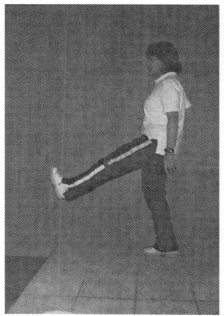 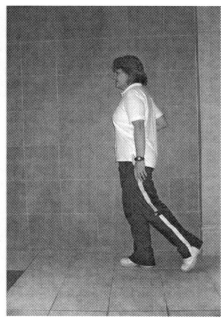

Straight Leg Raise

Technique: Tighten quadriceps, lock knee joint, and kick forward within a tolerable range of stretch, hold two seconds, then lower leg and kick back slightly to touch toe down. Keep opposing heel down while kicking other leg forward. Repetition: Start with 10-12 reps, and increase to 15, then 20. Two sets of 15 reps are sufficient. If you have sciatica and experience pain further down the leg with kicks, decrease reps or hold off altogether until this is comfortable. Adaptation: Try kicking in the middle of the pool, using only one or two barbells for balance. This requires greater balance and increases joint stability.

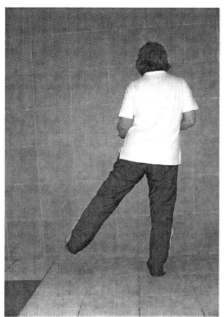
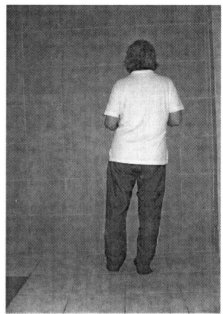

Hip Abduction

Technique: Hold onto side of pool and kick leg out, hold 2 seconds, then bring back in and touch ankles together. Be sure to lead with the side of your foot, even turning the foot in slightly into a pigeon-toed position. You do not have to kick out as far as your can—half of this range, approximately a 45-degree angle is sufficient.

Repetition: Start with 12 reps, increase to 15, then 20. Two sets of 15 reps (or 30 total) are plenty. Adaptation: If you have sciatica or a herniated disc, you may experience increased low back or buttock pain on the side with sciatica. Reduce the angle of the kicks, reduce the repetitions, or hold off altogether. Try this exercise using only barbells to help you balance versus holding onto the side of the pool.

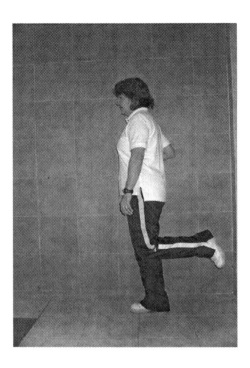

Hamstring Curl

Technique: Hold onto the side of the pool to stabilize yourself. Curl the lower leg and heel back and up toward your buttock. Do not let the upper leg come forward as you curl the lower leg. You can prevent this by placing the knees side by side. If you have arthritic knees or another knee problem, this exercise may be uncomfortable. This uses the back of the upper leg (hamstrings) while stretching out the front of the thigh (quadriceps). If the knee joint pain is too uncomfortable don't raise the heel as high and do 10 or less repetitions. Repetition: As tolerated if you have bad arthritic knees. Otherwise, start with 12, then 15, working up to 20 reps. Two sets of 15 repetitions total is sufficient. Adaptation: Kick in the middle of the pool, using barbells only to assist in balance.

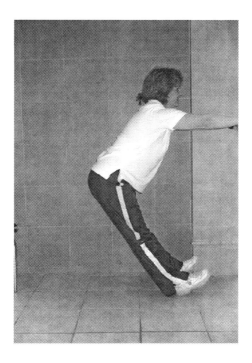

Heel-Toe Rocks

Technique: This is an excellent low back stretch and calf stretch. Hold onto the side of the pool or ladder, rock forward up on toes, then roll back on your heels as you lower yourself back, pressing the hips out and back until your shoulders are in the water. Now raise your toes up so you are only on your heels and holding on with your hands. Hold for a count of 5, sink back a little more, then pull up and back up onto toes, into an upright position. For chronic low back or stenotic backs, this is a wonderful stretch. Hold for much longer when you are back on your heels for relief. Repetition: Start with 12, work up to 15 or 20 repetitions; this is sufficient. The relief comes in holding the posture longer versus doing more repetitions. Adaptation: None

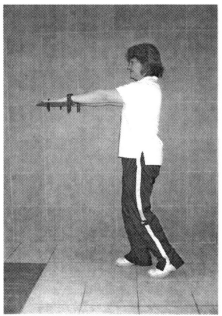 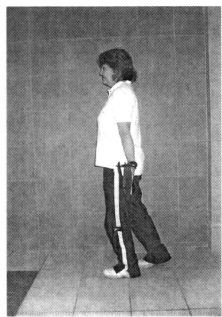

Paddle Exercise #1

Technique: Secure paddle with strap on the middle finger and wrist. Slightly stagger one foot in front of the other to help you counter-balance. Elbows are essentially locked in this exercise. Push palms down past the hips slightly, stop, and flip paddles with palms facing upward. Tighten abdominal muscles and push palms up toward the water's surface. Stop and flip paddles with palms facing down and repeat. Remember to flip the paddles at the top and bottom of the arm position each time. Keep abdominals and low back taut and this will help you not lose your balance. If you need extra stability for balance, start this by leaning against the pool wall. Work yourself off of the wall as soon as you can to better work on trunk strengthening and balance. Repetition: Start with 12 to 15 reps, work up to 20 and then two sets of 20 reps. You can even do this by time, doing it continuously for 2 to 4 minutes. Adaptation: In the next paddle exercises.

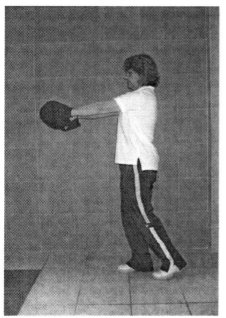 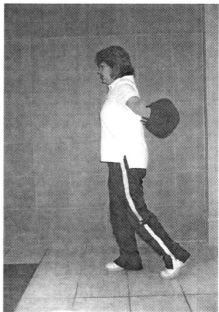

Paddle Exercise #2

Technique: Secure the paddle on the middle finger and at the wrist with the straps. Stagger your feet slightly so one foot is in front of the other. Do not have your feet more than shoulder width apart if possible. Palms and paddles are turned facing outward at chest high level. Elbows are essentially locked, arms stiff. Push arms back until they are slightly past the shoulders, remaining about chest high level. Stop and flip paddles so palms are now facing forward. Tighten abdominals to help maintain balance and bring hands forward as if clapping them together. Stop and flip paddles and repeat. Remember to go slightly past the shoulders and trunk; this helps you recruit and better isolate the abdominals. If you cannot keep your balance, move into shallower water. Repetition: Start with 12 to 15 reps, working up to 20 reps, and then two sets of 15 to 20 reps, if able. If this bothers your neck or shoulders move to shallower water, below chest level. Adaptation: None, this is a great exercise!

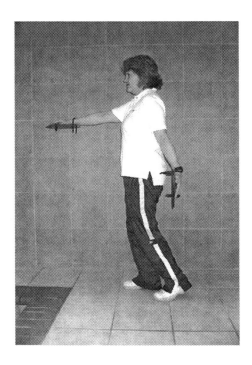

Paddle Exercise #3

Technique: Secure paddle to hand on middle finger and at the wrist. Stagger the feet, one foot slightly ahead of the other and feet about shoulder width apart. Elbows are essentially locked. One palm/arm is on top of the water, facing downward. The other arm is at the side of the hip, with the palm facing upward. Push one palm down, and push the palm facing up to the surface of the water. Stop and flip paddles; one palm is on top of the water facing down, the other arm is at the side of the hip, palm facing upward. Push down with the down palm, push up with the up palm. Stop and flip paddles. The key to this exercise is stopping before you flip your palms, otherwise forget it. This exercise works the deep muscles that rotate the spine. Repetition: Same as the other paddle exercises. Work up to 2 to 4 minutes ideally. Adaptation: None. If you have trouble with this one, just start slowly until you can get the rhythm. Remember, stop then flip.

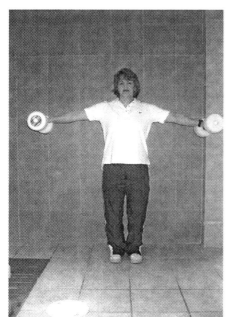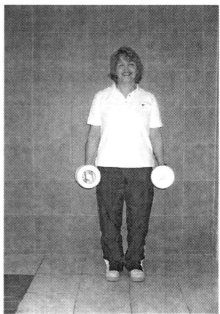

Barbell Exercise #1

Technique: Hold hand barbells out to the side in chest-high water. Elbows will be locked, feet shoulder-width apart, with knees slightly bent. Tighten abdominals and breathe out as you push the barbells under to the sides of your legs. Slowly let the barbells come to the surface and repeat again. Repetition: Start with 12 repetitions, then work up to 15, then 20. Two sets of 15 to 20 reps is sufficient. Adaptation: The resistance can be graded in this exercise, going light with open fan wheels to large foam barbells. To work more on balance you can do this exercise while standing on one leg, then switch to the other leg on the second set.

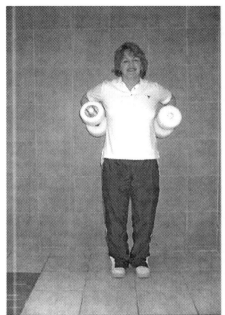 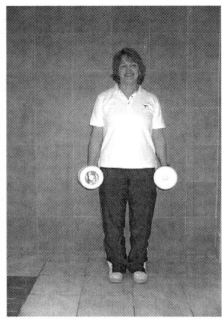

Barbell Push-Downs

Technique: Start in chest-high water. Place barbells next to your sides, with barbells at chest level. Feet are shoulder-width apart with knees slightly bent. Exhale as you push the barbells under, keeping them close to your sides as you push down. Relax and let the barbells slowly return to the water's surface. Repeat. Repetition: 15 to 20 reps. Work up as you want. Two sets of 15 should be sufficient. Adaptation: You may stand on one leg if you want to challenge your balance. If you have arthritis or tendonitis of the shoulder, this exercise may be uncomfortable. Skip this one if it bothers your shoulders.

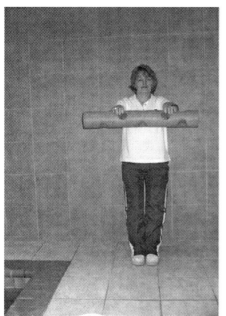 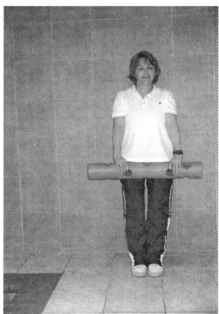

Ab Crunches

Technique: You can use a medium size ball, hand barbell(s), or a long single barbell or foam roll for this exercise. The resistance is harder in deeper water or by using a denser object to push under water. A medium size ball will be harder to push under than a triangle size hand barbell. Place back against pool wall or rail. Slightly bend knees; this takes the legs out of the exercise so you cannot use them for leverage but instead you isolate and use the abdominals and shoulder muscles. You will be in chest high (or slightly less) water. You should be leaning against the wall, knees bent, shoulders back. Push ball (or barbell) under to the top of the thighs, hold 5 seconds, then let the ball slowly come up; don't let the ball pop up out of the water, because it will. Elbows are locked on this exercise. This is a great stabilizing exercise for the arms and for the trunk (isometric ab crunches!). Repetition: 15 to 20 reps. Work up to your tolerance. Adaptation: The denser the object, the greater the resistance, so you can progressively upgrade this exercise.

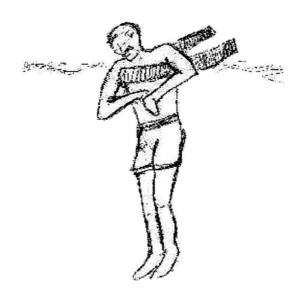

Hangin' Out

Technique: This exercise is literally hanging in the deep end of the pool to dis-
tract the spine, allowing arthritic joints to breathe, or distraction off of an irritated nerve root or disc. For many people, this exercise offers tremendous relief.
In cases of really acute sciatica or a disc, the deep water traction many not be tolerated too well or for too long. If you experience leg pain, move to shallow water.
Repetition: We have our clientele stay in the deep end 10 minutes on average
unless they get really good relief then they can stay up to 20 minutes. Adaptation:
Floating on a raft is non-weight bearing and supportive, but you don't get the
vertical distraction of the spine and joints, so I recommend deep water hanging.
Also, for arthritic hips or knees, we sometimes add a 2.5 to 5 pound ankle weight,
but not greater than 5 pounds. One must be more careful using weights for low
back pain. If the condition is osteoarthritis or degenerative disc disease, weights
will probably be fine. I do not recommend using weights with a sciatic condition.
The slightest increase in tension on the nerve can easily inflame an already angry
nerve root. Remember, as a rule, be cautious initially using weights and 5 pounds
is usually maximum.

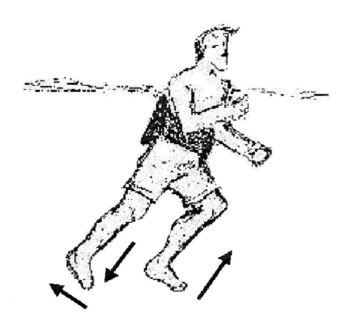

Deep Water Jog

Technique: This exercise works on trunk strengthening and stabilization. Jogging in a vertical posture creates 12 times more resistance, so this almost doubles what you can do on land because of increased work output. Fifteen minutes of continuous moderate paced jogging in the water equates to about 30 minutes of jogging on land. This is a wonderful alternative for runners experiencing back pain. You unload the spine and lower extremity joints while working on strength and endurance. The correct posture for this exercise is an erect trunk, slightly leaning forward with no bend at the waist. The knees do not come up high, not past a 45 degree angle. You strike the heel down and back. I liken it to riding an unicycle or pushing a scooter; do not let the knees come up like you are riding a bicycle because this takes the trunk and low back completely out of the exercise. You are going to feel like you are running in slow motion, up an incline, or through jello. This exercise is not about speed but about the correct posture. This is a mild to moderate cardiovascular exercise, but most important, it is a trunk strengthening exercise, working upper back, abdominals, postural muscles of the back, the gluteals and hip flexors. The momentum of the exercise is dictated by the arms.

Keep the hands in a loose fist to prevent your using them like paddles; make your body push through the water, don't pull it with your arms. Stick with this. It is awkward at first, but after several attempts, you will suddenly find the rhythm. The mistake most people make is bringing the knees up too high. Remember the leg strikes down and back, like pushing along on a scooter. Repetition: Start with 5 minutes to test the tolerance of your low back; this is a fairly high level exercise for the back. Gradually build up your time, never increasing more than 5 minutes a session. Do at least 2 to 3 sessions at a certain duration before increasing the time; don't increase each time or you will get yourself in trouble. Adaptation: Once you work up to 15 to 20 minutes of jogging consistently without any problems, you may want to bump up your program. You can get aqua-jogging shoes made of dense foam. They are light-weight but require you to work/kick harder so you may get more of a cardiovascular work out. Remember first and foremost, this is a back strengthening exercise before it is a cardiovascular workout (in this context). Always respect the back and work to your tolerance, otherwise you'll be taking several days off for overdoing it.

FLEXIBILITY STRETCHES

The importance of flexibility in combating back pain cannot be overemphasized. When you have a normal (or near normal) length of a muscle, it allows for greater joint articulation and better joint efficiency and mechanics. Don't you think that is important in joints that are being compromised by degenerative changes? All of the lower extremity stretches included in the water exercise section involve all the major joints. In the event that you don't have access to a pool for whatever reason, I have included the land versions of these same stretches.

Stretching the quadriceps, hamstrings, hip flexors (psoas) and hip rotators (piriformis) is important to ensure functional mobility of the pelvis, which indirectly affects the lumbar spine. Our sedentary lifestyle and professions contribute to shortened hamstrings, quadriceps, hip flexors and hip rotators and extensors. Another thing that contributes to shortened muscle groups involved with the pelvis would be the use of a cane or walker.

Ideally, flexibility is enhanced when stretching is done 3 to 4 times a week. Sometimes when my back is bothering me, I will spend 5 to 10 minutes going through the four stretches I have included and it eases my back pain considerably. Gains in flexibility are enhanced in water. If you can't do them in water, they can be done on land. If you are unable to get in the water, for example when you are traveling. Consistency is the key. Dedicate yourself to stretching 5 to 10 minutes, 3 to 4 times a week. You will see a change **and** feel it.

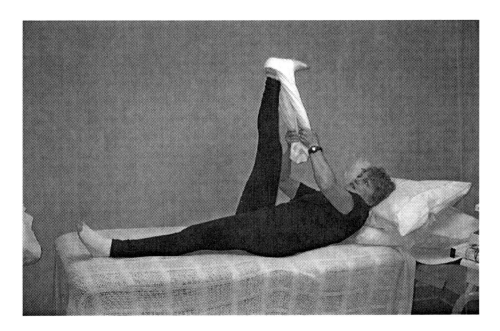

Hamstring (Towel) Stretch

Technique: Lying flat to stretch the hamstring protects the low back, particularly the disc and sciatic nerve. The other knees is bent also to protect the back while stretching the hamstring. The stretch in the picture is more aggressive because both legs are straight. Initially, start with the bent knee when stretching the opposite leg. Place the towel across the heel—if you place it on the ball of the foot it also stretches the calf, which is a more aggressive stretch on the sciatic nerve. Start with the knee on the stretching leg slightly bent with the towel over the heel. Slowly straighten the leg before pulling toward the head. Straightening the leg alone will stretch the hamstring within a tolerable limit. After you straighten the leg and lock the knee, hold this for 20 seconds. After holding this, if you feel the muscle relax some, gradually pull it up toward the head, hold 20 seconds, then gradually relax the leg. Repetition: Repeat 3 to 4 times on each leg, holding the stretch for 30 to 60 seconds. Adaptation: Work first on locking out the knee versus pulling the leg up high. Allow the muscle to accommodate to the stretch. 90 degree to 100 degree angle is a normal and sufficient range for the hamstring.

Use caution with the hamstring stretch. It is most effective when there is _no_ leg pain. If leg pain is present, it is best to avoid this stretch until the leg pain has significantly improved or resolved. This stretch can potentially aggravate an acutely irritated nerve. Use caution.

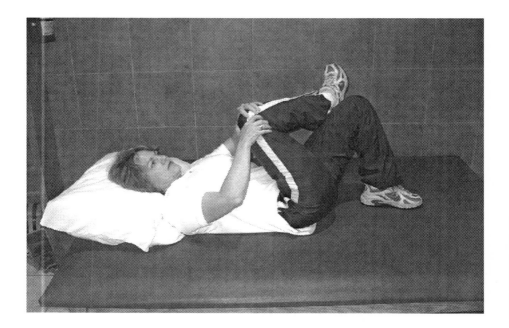

Piriformis Stretch

Technique: Lie flat, crossing one leg over the other, with the ankle resting on the opposite knee. Feet should be placed slightly wider than the hips, if tolerable. Grab on the outside of the knee (or under the knee if more comfortable) of the crossed leg. Pull gently toward the opposite shoulder, in a diagonal line. Pull in and hold for 20 seconds. After you feel the muscle relax slightly, pull in further toward opposite shoulder. Hold for another 15 to 20 seconds. Slowly release tension for a few seconds and repeat. Repetition: Repeat 3 to 4 times on each leg, holding the stretch 30 to 60 seconds. Adaptation: Keep the ankle on the knee and the feet at the width of the hips or slightly wider for a better stretch. If this increases buttock or leg pain, do not do this one as it puts tension at the nerve root.

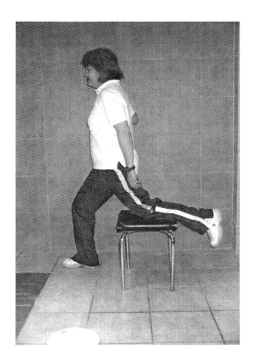

Psoas (Hip Flexor) Stretch

Technique: This stretch is excellent for people who sit a lot, use a cane or walker, or tend to walk slightly stooped because you have shortened hip flexors because of these postures. Use a chair or surface about that height. Place knee on surface and place opposite leg and foot in front of the knee on the chair. This is the initial stretch. Now slightly bend the knee of the standing leg and let the hips go forward, putting further stretch on the psoas. Hold this stretch for 20 to 30 seconds, release, then press hips forward again, bending the knee of the standing leg. You may need to use the wall or another chair to help you balance if your psoas is really tight. Repetition: Repeat 3 to 4 times on one leg, then switch legs. Hold each stretch for 30 to 60 seconds. Adaptation: The further forward you put the standing leg, the greater the stretch. Keep an upright posture through this stretch.

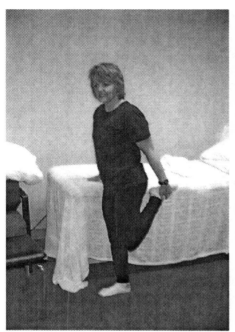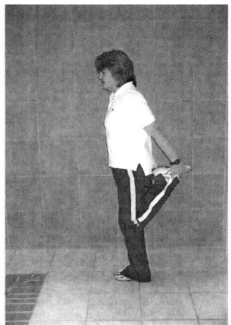

Quadriceps Stretch

Technique: This exercise may be done standing but may be more comfortable for stenotic backs in a side-lying posture. In either position, grab the front of the foot, bend the knee, keeping the thigh straight, and gently pull the heel toward the buttock. If you cannot reach your heel, wrap a towel around the ankle and pull the ends of the short hand towel. Try to keep the trunk straight and don't allow bending at the waist or hip. Pull until you feel a good stretch on the front of the thigh and hold this for 20 seconds. If you feel the muscle relax, pull the heel in further toward the buttock and hold another 15 seconds. Try not to let the hip flex, but maintain an upright posture. Repetition: Repeat 3 to 4 stretches on one leg, then switch. Hold each stretch for 30 to 60 seconds. Adaptation: May be done in side-lying position for greater comfort. Use a hand towel around the ankle if you cannot reach your foot.

EQUIPMENT RESOURCES

Finally, you are sold on water therapy as a means to manage and correct low back pain and its disabling effects. You have the illustrated exercises in sequence, you have found a pool or have a pool, and you're ready to go. Yes, you can use gallon milk jugs and saucers to supplement your program; they will work. However, I know what a difference proper equipment can make to a program and I urge you to buy a few inexpensive pieces and I will tell you where to get them.

Water exercise may well become the primary means of exercise for many of you so make it as effective as it possibly can be. I also have listed a company that carries ergonomic furniture and other excellent accessories for the workplace to help get you comfortably through your day. All of these companies have been in the business of water exercise or back-related products for years and are highly reputable.

My recommended equipment list:

1.   Texas Swim Shop
     Houston, TX
     713-723-0910

     This locally owned family business has served my clients and Texas swim teams for decades. They carry all different kinds of equipment and if they don't have it in stock, they can get it right away. Don't hesitate to call them.

2.   Sprint-Rothhamer or Rothhamer International
     Santa Monica, CA
     800-235-2156
     www.sprintaquatics.com

     This international pool products/exercise company carries a vast array of all swim needs. They have water exercise equipment, safety aids, and a variety of water-related videos, books and aerobic music.

3.   Hydro-Tone
     16691 Gothard Street, Suite M
     Huntington Beach, CA 92647

800-622-TONE; 714-848-8284
www.hydro-tone.com

This national company carries all types of water exercise equipment in addition to water-related books, videos and aerobic music.

4. Aqua-Jogger
    4048 West 1st Avenue, Unit B
    Eugene, OR 97402-9391
    800-922-9544; 541-484-2454

This company exploded on the water exercise scene years ago with the original Aqua-Jogger belt, with many knock-offs to follow their lead. This company specializes in deep-water jogging products, including videos, charts, belts and aqua-jogging shoes. The aqua-jogging shoes are great if you find you like the deep water jogging. The aqua-shoes fit comfortably over your feet and secure with a Velcro strap in back. The shoes make you work harder by requiring you to kick harder and overcome increased resistance. We use these with the clients who have mastered deep water jogging and **know** they can tolerate it without increased symptoms and want to notch up their workout.

5. Relax The Back Store
    800-222-5728
    www.relaxtheback.com

This national company has a comprehensive selection of products, including ergonomic furniture, chairs and work-related products. Their products are of the finest quality and are guaranteed, making their asking price worthwhile. The have some excellent seat cushions, back supports for the work chair and car, and comfortable pillows. I really like their **self-inflating** travel pillow, about $40-50 dollars. This pillow rolls up to fit into a purse or briefcase to answer your travel quandaries concerning lack of back support in planes, meetings or rental cars.

Also try:

> Excel Sports Science, Inc.
> NZ Manufacturing, Inc.
> Speedo, Inc.

Equipment Needs

I recommend getting the following pieces of equipment for your water therapy program.

Barbells

These lightweight foam barbells come in varying levels of resistance: light, medium, and heavy. Most of you can use medium to heavy/large. The wider the barbell ring, the greater the resistance. Remember you can vary the resistance by moving shallower or deeper (more resistance) in the pool. Therefore, I think it is better to get medium to large barbells and use them as you are able to do more.

Aqua-jogger makes a triangle barbell which works well as an addition to your water-walking. You don't want so much resistance that it throws you off balance. Remember the focus of the program is trunk stabilization and control. Fit the equipment to the purpose of the exercise.

Paddles

This is the most important piece of equipment and can easily be taken on trips. These paddles come in small, medium, large, and extra-large. Most of you will use at least a large, maybe a medium if you have any kind of shoulder problems. Most of our clients, including our seniors, graduate to the extra-large swim paddles as they master trunk control. Originally, paddles were designed to help swimmers learn better stroke technique and build their arms and upper back. Remember, moving paddles faster increases the resistance in the exercises.

Ab Crunches

An array of equipment can be used to do the ab crunch exercise. You can use a single barbell, which is what we start many of our ladies on, and increase it accordingly. You may use a rough surfaced ball, like a dimple ball or tether ball, but don't get one that is too big because it will be harder to control. We upgrade our clients from a single long buoy, to a double or triple bar buoy. These will most likely be referred to as swim-aids or teaching aids (used with kids learning to swim). You can also use the large, thick noodles that are available at most large retail outlet stores. Abdominal exercises are important in building trunk strength and stability.

Jog-Belts

There are several types of belts on the market and they all basically function on an equal basis. The belts come in small, medium and large and these are related to a weight range. Aqua-jogger does make a belt that is thicker if you need more buoyancy. Most of us don't have problem with buoyancy, however!

Ankle-Weights

Waterproof ankle weights are available and heavily utilized in our program. If you are going to use weights, get the waterproof. Otherwise, regular weights turn hard and become inflexible; they don't work. Weight dimensions are about 1, 2.5, 3, 5, 7.5 and 10 pounds. We use the 2.5, 5, and 7.5 pound weights. They won't feel as heavy in the water so get at least the 2 to 3 pound weights. Ten-pound weights are probably too much for the exercises, but can be used with deep-water traction, although we find the 7.5 pound weights to be sufficient here. Be sure you can tolerate the deep-water traction 10 minutes without increased symptoms before you use weights with deep-water traction.

Getting Through the Day With Back Pain

IT'S ALL IN THE MIND

Don't get nervous; I'm not calling you "crazy" or a "fake." However, managing back pain successfully really is all in your mind. It is called planning. You have learned about postures and the loads they generate on the spine. You have learned about creep and how its onset occurs within 90 minutes. Creep is also affected by factors such as age, genetics, previous injuries, level of fitness, and disease, to name a few. You have also learned that as you recover, you operate within a window of tolerance.

This window of tolerance will change as you recover, but one must always factor in activities of everyday life when defining the level of loading tolerance. Once you know what pushes the load tolerance to the high end, you can control it, for the most part. There will be activities that aggravate your back pain, as well as activities that relieve it. Think about your day and plan it accordingly to better manage your back pain. Let's look at some patients who successfully learned these principles.

Ruth came in with a flare-up of sciatica, which she had been dealing with for two years. She had spinal stenosis, with poor standing and walking tolerance. She and her husband were embarking on a preplanned (and pre-purchased) two-week trip to Europe. I wondered if she would make it. Three weeks later she returned and announced she had a wonderful time with little to manageable back pain. This is how she did it. She brought a lightweight camping stool that folded up like an umbrella. When they went on a walking tour of various museums, she simply pulled out her stool and sat whenever she needed. This relieved her back pain. If she didn't feel like she could climb stairs, she didn't. If she did a lot of walking one day, the next day she scheduled little to nothing. She knew how to plan her day to minimize her back and leg pain.

Many of our clients schedule their lodging at a hotel that has a pool or workout facility when they travel. They do their pool program or stretching to counteract whatever paces their back has been through that day.

Maria was a writer. She had struggled two years with various types of intervention for her back pain, all unsuccessful. She had a publishing deadline and a writer's workshop coming up in a four months and was fearful she couldn't make either of them. She did. She started doing the pool program at her home and managed her pain by sitting only limited amounts of time while writing. She came to understand creep and the fact that her window of sitting tolerance was limited. By managing her sitting, breaking up her day with unloading by getting in the pool or lying down, her window of tolerance gradually started improving.

She learned that certain activities exceeded her window of tolerance, like driving or sitting too much in the car. She planned her days and managed her pain. I did get a postcard from her when she was at her writer's workshop. She was hiking daily and writing up a storm. By respecting the process, she changed her window of tolerance—something you too can do.

Let me comment briefly on planning your day by referencing your window of loading tolerance. Sitting is going to be a big challenge for many of you. Your tolerance for sitting may be 15 minutes or two hours. Let's say it's two hours. What if you go to dinner and have to wait 20 minutes for a table? Guess what? The meter is running. If you go to the bar and have a drink while you wait—stand up! Walk to the restroom; do something besides sit. If dinner (including the wait) takes an hour, that leaves out a movie, which would be another 90 to 120 minutes (minimum) of sitting. If you really want to go to that movie, don't do dinner. Sometimes you may be able to do dinner and a movie, but know this is pushing the upper end of the window. Don't try it often. Be respectful of your back.

If you go to the movie and know you can sit only 45-60 minutes, get the aisle seat. Then, walk to the back of the theater and stand a while, stretch—just move. Break up that process of creep. If you go to a conference or meeting, sit in the back. Get up and move around as needed. All of these tricks really, really work. Think about the activities of your day and plan accordingly. Give your back a break as much as you can, and it will give you a break in return.

DAILY LIFE—HELPFUL HINTS

As you have now learned, everyday life can be hard on the back! I'm talking everyday life—driving the car, cleaning the house, taking care of kids and pets, sitting through business meetings, flying, walking long distances in the airport or parking lots, even cooking—all of these acts of daily living can be overwhelming to someone dealing with back pain. Things that you never knew could be challenging, even harmful to your back now seem to be so. Is there any help out there? Yes, there is. I wanted to include this chapter to shed light on everyday tasks and how to better manage, even avoid some things that may not be so great for your back now that back pain requires so much more of your consideration and planning. Let's look at some areas of concern.

Driving

Driving can be a big irritant to many of you—especially if you are in the car a considerable amount of time. Studies have shown that "men (or women) who spend at least 50% of their work time driving a motor vehicle are three times more likely to develop a herniated disc" than those individuals who do not drive for a living. I have seen plenty of bus drivers or traveling salespersons as patients over the years. What makes driving so hazardous? The vibration produced on the spine, as well as the increased loading on the lumbar discs in the seated position overwhelms the discs over a period of time and leads to the degenerated state. Dr. Augustus White also proposed that the vibration of the spine, the added load in sitting on the spine and the "limited variety of optional sitting positions available to the driver may result in a predisposition to disc herniation." (White and Panjabi 1978, 279) What can you do to combat this?

Sitting/Riding in the Car

Fortunately, car manufacturers have addressed this problem fairly well in recent years. The pneumatic lumbar support is now available in most cars. I don't know about you, but after a while I have to keep adding more air to my lumbar support. Is it possible that lumbar car supports suffer "creep" just like you and me? My point is this. Make sure your lumbar support is firm or it really is not going to help much. There are lumbar rolls of various sizes and firmness on the market, as well as car pillows. My support actually has a hard shell base that extends to the upper back and has the lumbar support built in. There is something that will work "just right" for you. Get something comfortable so you will use it consistently.

Seat Position

Kelsey and Hardy did a study (1975) that determined the predisposition toward disc herniation for those individuals that drive at least 50% or more as part of their job. This same study also showed "the use of armrests as well as a lumbar support reduced intradiscal pressure." Adequate thigh support, the depth of the seat, can help off load low back pressures to the discs, too. A prime example of an inadequate seat would be most airplane seats. Most have no lumbar support and hit you about mid thigh. Just like riding in the car, there is very limited wiggle room—your knees are against the seat in front of you and your elbows are to your sides. If you travel much, I'm sure backaches are familiar to you. Help is on the way.

Studies have shown that a seat reclined to 120 degrees (with 90 degrees being upright) decreases the amount of disc pressure significantly. Next time you get into the car or plane, use a lumbar support and slightly recline the seat back to 120 degrees to decrease pressure on the lumbar spine. Otherwise, when sitting try to have your feet in contact with the floor and hips and knees flexed to 90 degrees. Don't have your car seat so far back that you are practically sliding down in the seat to reach the gas pedal. These tricks, as simple as they are, really do help!

Lifting—Push/Pull

Between the ages of 40 to 60 years, the compressive load tolerance to the lumbar vertebrae decline about 50 percent (White and Panjabi 1978, 30) Your body is changing; it can't do as much physically so you can't be as carefree and reckless as you work around the house or in the yard. If you are moving a long water hose from the side yard to the front, don't drag it. Face forward and pull it behind you. Don't drag a bag of potting soil as you backpedal your way to the flowerbed. Place it in a wagon or wheelbarrow and push it to where you're going; this way the load is in front of you and you maintain your spine in an upright posture versus being bent over at the waist. The vertebral unit is more strained in flexion or at some inclination. "The motion segment provides greater resistance to failure when the loads are applied centrally." (White and Panjabi 1978, 39) This supports the long preached principle of lifting with your spine straight rather than flexed. Bend your knees not your back, and keep the load as close as possible to you as you lift. Remember, too, push—don't pull. "Studies comparing pushing and pulling and the amounts of intra-thoracic and intra-abdominal pressures revealed pushing produced less loading of the spine than pulling." (White and Panjabi 1978, 352)

Weight

Being significantly overweight greatly increases the wear and tear on the spine and accelerates the break down of tissue and joints. A large abdomen is the same as carrying an external object that weighs that 30, 40, 50 or 60 pounds of extra fat you are carrying on your trunk. Your center of gravity is located approximately 1-1/2" to 2" below your navel. A large abdomen puts an anterior shift or pull on the lumbar spine, which puts increased wear and tear on the joints of the spine.

"Obesity greatly increases both the direct vertical compressive load on the spine and the anteriorly acting loads, which create very large joint reaction forces" (White and Panjabi 1978, 334). Translation—the additional load coming from fatty tissue increases the compressive load down through the spine. The heavy abdomen also creates load in front (or anterior) to the spine which causes the joints of the spine to work harder to counteract this forward pull on the spine. It all leads to wear and tear on the joints which will lead to osteoarthritis of the spine. Don't let your weight get out of control. It just accelerates the aging of your body, overall, not to mention the additional stress on the cardiovascular system.

Walking

Two exercises that have been perpetuated over the years as being important in addressing low back pain are walking and the sit-up. Walking with a slight arm swing has proven to be beneficial. Strolling is not beneficial to the spine because with frequent stopping, such as window shopping, the spine is subjected to frequent static loading. Faster walking with some arm swinging offers some light loading of the spine with muscle activation in the trunk through the arm swinging. The momentum of the arm swing helps decrease the load through the spine.

However, not everyone can tolerate walking. Those individuals suffering from acute sciatica or spinal stenosis cannot tolerate walking any significant distances. In these cases, one can use a recumbent bike, which employs a more tolerant position of flexion. Or, one can do a combined workout on the treadmill and recumbent bike.

Sit-ups

Haven't you always heard that strong abdominal muscles help support the lumbar spine? That is true, but it is not exactly an endorsement of the sit-up. According to Stuart McGill, the acclaimed biomechanical engineer and researcher, "the goal is to challenge muscle at the appropriate levels but in a way that spares the spine." Too many back sufferers are given exercises that actually "exceed the tolerance of their compromised tissues." (McGill 2002, 104)

Dr. Augustus White goes further in disputing the sit-up as advantageous in the rehabilitation of back pain. "The sit-up exercise is contra-indicated in individuals with degenerative lumbar disc disease. The loads exerted on the lumbar spine while doing a sit-up are comparable to those caused by improperly lifting 44 lbs." (White and Panjabi 1978, 306) I don't know about you, but I know I don't want to lift 44 lbs. wrong, so I am not going to do something that is comparable. Isometric contractions of the abdominal musculature are beneficial and commonly referred to as stabilization exercises. The muscle groups of the trunk contract but don't really involve any motion. There are several stabilization exercises included in the water therapy section where you use the trunk muscles without actually flexing or extending the spine. Dr. Stuart McGill simply stated that "sit-ups should not be performed at all by most people." (McGill 2002, 105)

Sex

Have you given up on it? Just too painful and frustrating to find a comfortable (even tolerable) position? There is hope; you don't have to give up this part of your life. It is just going to take some patience and tinkering to find what is going to work for you and your partner. There is a wonderful booklet available called "Sex and Back Pain." It is available through OPTP at 1-800-367-7393. I recommend it to all my patients and encourage you to give it a look before you completely give up on sex.

CONCLUSION

Hopefully you have learned more about your back after working your way through this book. With aging comes several other factors that figure into the healing process and preventative phase. Previous injury, state of overall health, age chronologically and physiologically, weight and degree of fitness are significant contributors to back pain, to name just a few.

You have learned of insidious biomechanical workings of the body known as load, creep and window of tolerance. Understanding that these workings in the body are always taking place, and that they are altered with injury and aging, helps you better accommodate them in the healing phase and beyond that into the maintenance phase.

When you are healing from injury or disuse, there are stages you go through to get the best results possible to get back into the mainstream of life. The stages of rehabilitation progress sequentially through the areas of flexibility, endurance, strength and coordination. By building upon each stage, the body heals more effectively and builds more joint stability as a means of injury (or re-injury) prevention.

Staying out of back pain requires two things. First, you must be aware of your daily activities and how they impact your back in relation to your individual history, and then plan accordingly. This daily reflection includes activities of daily life, work related demands, and leisure and exercise pursuits. With any major change in lifestyle, daily planning is central to keeping any gains you make. This is true whether it is weight loss, abstinence from alcohol or smoking, or living with a physical impairment—in this case, back pain. What things make your back better? What activities definitely aggravate your back pain? Plan accordingly and make changes where they are necessary and where you can.

Finally, you must have exercise as part of your daily life if you want to stay out of the cycle of back pain. Due to injury, disease, age, weight or other such factors, you must build your endurance and strength to aid degenerating discs or arthritic joints. Whereas conventional exercise may have failed you in the past, you can now accommodate your pain and physical limitations through water exercise. Eliminating the compressive forces of gravity enable you to more comfortably address losses in flexibility, endurance, strength and coordination. It also does wonders for your mental outlook and confidence. Once you find you can move safely in the water without much pain or likelihood of injury, then you do just that—move. This restores your confidence as you progress in your water therapy program. Whether you have to stay in the water to exercise or you are able to move on isn't the focus. The focus is to get you moving and on the road to recovery, to reclaiming your life. The water will always be a place you can come to, or come back to, should your back pain return.

And return it will. However, you no longer have to be a victim or prisoner of your back. Living harmoniously, even contently, with back pain is an achievable goal. All of this is possible to different degrees for each of us. You must be consistent. There will be episodes of overdoing it, but eventually you learn your parameters—what is going to work or not work for you. You are ultimately the key ingredient here. I encourage you to participate and be very involved in the decisions concerning your health. You will be happier when you are central to all of these decisions. It is your responsibility to be in charge if you want results. I wish you the best as you reclaim your life from back pain. It is possible.

REFERENCES

1. American College of Sports Medicine. 1978. *Position statement on the recommended quantity and quality of exercise for healthy adults.* Indianapolis, American College of Sports Medicine.

2. American College of Sports Medicine. "Position statement on the recommended quantity and quality of exercise for development and maintaining cardiorespiratory and muscular fitness in healthy adults." *Med Sci Sports 22* (1990): 265-274.

3. Baechle, Thomas, and Earle, Roger. 1994. *Essentials of strength training and conditioning.* Human Kinetics, NSCA.

4. Bogduk, Nikolai. 1997. *Clinical anatomy of the lumbar spine and sacrum.* 3rd Edition. Philadelphia: Elsevier Ltd.

5. Bortz, WM. "The disuse syndrome." *West J. Med 141* (1984): 691-694.

6. Calliet, Rene, M.D. 1995. *Low back pain syndrome.* Edition 5, F.A. Davis Company.

7. Corrigan, Brian, and Matland, G.D. 1993. *Practical orthopedic medicine.* Butterworth, Heinemann Publishing.

8. DeFranca, George. 1996. *Pelvic locomotor dysfunction.* Aspen Publishers.

9. Fredette, Denise. 1998. Chapter 54 "Recommendations for flexibility and range of motion," in *ACSM's Resource Manual: Guidelines for Exercise Testing and Prescription.* 3rd ed. Edited by Jeffrey L. Roitman. New York: Lippincott, Williams and Wilkins Publishing, 456-464.

10. Goldstein, Trudy Sandler. 1995. *Functional rehabilitation in orthopedics.* Aspen Publishers.

11. Grelsamer M.D., Ronald, and Loebl, Suzanne. 1997. *The Columbia Presbyterian Osteoarthritis Handbook.* Macmillan.

12. Kaplan M.D., Frederick S. 1987. *Osteoporosis: pathophysiology and prevention.* Clinical Symposia 39(1). Summit, NJ: Ciba-Geigy Corporation.

13. Kazarian, L.E. "Creep characteristics of the human spinal column." *Orthop Clin North Am* 6:3 (1975): 3-18.

14. Kirkaldy-Willis, W.H. 1983. *Managing low back pain.* Churchill-Livingstone.

15. Lewis, Carole, and Bottomley, J. 1994. *Geriatric physical therapy.* Appleton & Lange.

16. Liebenson, Craig. 1996. *Rehabilitation of the spine.* Lippincott, Williams & Wilkins.

17. McGill, Stuart. 2002. *Low back disorders.* Human Kinetics.

18. Nachemson, A.L. "The lumbar spine, an orthopedic challenge." *Spine 1* (1976): 59.

19. Porterfield, James, and DeRosa, Carl. 1991. *Mechanical low back pain.* W.B. Saunders Company.

20. Slovik M.D., David. 2000. *Boosting bone strength: A guide to preventing and treating osteoporosis.* Harvard Health Publications.

21. White III, Augustus, and Panjabi, Manohar. 1978. *Clinical biomechanics of the spine.* J.B. Lippincott Company.

22. White, Martha. 1995. *Water exercise.* Human Kinetics.

23. Whiting, Wm, and Zernicke, Ronald. 1998. *Biomechanics of musculoskeletal injury.* Human Kinetics.

24. Winston, Leland. 1995. *Water exercise.* Human Kinetics.

0-595-32887-3

CPSIA information can be obtained at www.ICGtesting.com
Printed in the USA
LVOW13s0300270813

349767LV00001B/66/A

9 780595 328871